Challenging Pregnancy

CHALLENGING PREGNANCY

(*A Journey through*
the Politics and Science
of Healthcare
in America)

Genevieve Grabman

UNIVERSITY OF IOWA PRESS, IOWA CITY

University of Iowa Press, Iowa City 52242
Copyright © 2022 by Genevieve Grabman
uipress.uiowa.edu

ISBN 978-1-60938-815-7 (pbk)
ISBN 978-1-60938-816-4 (ebk)

Printed in the United States of America
Design by April Leidig

Printed on acid-free paper

Cataloging-in-Publication data is on file
with the Library of Congress.

To my twins,
and to my doctors who saved them

(*Contents*)

(*Acknowledgments*)

These pages about twins, science, and politics evoke the memory of Dan Thomas, my copy editor, friend, and Oxford comma opponent. Just before this book went into production, Dan died of an inadvertent overdose of a prescription medication he took as ordered. Other countries warn of this drug's dangers, but the United States does not. Perhaps the medication adversely reacted with Dan's other prescriptions; we will never know because his care was not coordinated across his many doctors and for his many medications. Good health policy is for all of us, women and men alike. RIP, Dan.

I also thank my agent, John W. Wright, who weathered New York City's COVID-19 tsunami in early 2020. I appreciate the risk you took to help me while simultaneously trying to maintain your health.

Appreciation is due to Meredith T. Stabel, my editor at the University of Iowa Press, and my exacting and speedy peer reviewers, Kathryn Marko, Cara Tenenbaum, and Thomas Pinckert. Any errors you find are my own and occurred despite the hard work of this expert team.

Finally, I am grateful to medical illustrator Myrthe Boijmans; UZ Leuven professor Jan Deprest; Medscape Drugs & Diseases manager Kathy Roarty; and Taylor & Francis for permitting me to use their beautiful artwork in this book. A few finely rendered pictures explained twin-to-twin transfusion syndrome more clearly than I could in more than two hundred pages. Thank you.

(*Author's Note*)

This work is a series of essays, vignettes really, about the science and politics of healthcare in today's America. The stories are arranged around my 2015 pregnancy with twins, a gestation that went sideways from its very inception but that turned out mostly well in the end. The credit and my eternal gratitude go to the scientists and doctors involved; a dedication to one appears in the chapter, "Blighted Ovum." No thanks are owed to the employer, hospital, local, or federal politicians who would have interposed themselves between my physicians and me.

To save my very young children from nevertheless inevitable future embarrassment, I have changed their names in this work. All other details about my kids are true and accurate, including that I fought hard for them because I love them and want the very best, productive, happy lives for them. Because I am an attorney who always fears lawsuits, I also do not identify by name the doctors who cared for me. Other information about these doctors is likewise honestly rendered, as are copies of my communications with them.

I would like to address openly my uses of "female" and "woman" when discussing research on pregnancy. Pregnancies are borne by people other than those identifying as female or women. I wish to include all people in my discussion of the scientific and political barriers to pregnancy. The overarching theme of this book is that decisions—and the politics of decision-making about health-related matters, such as reproduction, pregnancy, and the postnatal period—affect everyone. To exclude anyone would be to create yet another obstacle to reproductive healthcare, and this discipline already has barriers aplenty, especially for people of color and non-gender-conforming individuals. But the adverse conditions of pregnancy I discuss, twin-to-twin transfusion syndrome (TTTS) and selective intrauterine growth restriction (sIUGR) are, blessedly, exceedingly rare. What data exist for these conditions are collected from pregnant people whose biological sex is reported as "female" and whose gender expression is described as "women." In the four years I spent researching this work, I never encountered studies about TTTS or sIUGR in nonfemale populations. And, until very recently, the study of maternal health focused wholly on the effect of pregnancy, including the prenatal and postpartum periods, on women's health.

My intent is to report correctly the scientific data for the conditions I describe. If the study populations were female, I so state. I have endeavored to use more inclusive terms wherever possible when discussing the political ramifications of pregnancy. When deliberating science or politics' effect on healthcare related to pregnancy and childbirth, I have employed the expression "maternal health" because that is how the discipline is most typically characterized.

I too wish to explain my discussion of race, especially the maternal and reproductive health outcomes of Black and white people, in an account of science and politics. Seemingly race-neutral health policies and procedures are applied to all pregnant patients, resulting in much worse outcomes for Black women. It may not be the intent of health providers to discriminate against Black people or to treat them differently from any other patient. But the racial gap in the maternal mortality and morbidity rates for Black and white women indicates a disparate impact of ostensibly unbiased care. Shining a light on this problem helps in pursuing its resolution.

You may be reading this book not for its exposition of the politics of pregnancy but rather as a how-to manual. Perhaps you are pregnant with twins or, God love you, your twin pregnancy is complicated by TTTS, sIUGR, or both. The references for each chapter contain links to every study I consulted. Throughout the work, I explain that not all studies are equal, and some are too small or designed too poorly to be relied on. Put into practice the suggestions I give for analyzing studies, especially those reported in the popular press. Read any research with a jaundiced eye and seek information from the gold standard of investigations: a randomized, controlled, clinical trial involving many participants who are a representative sample of those who experience the condition studied.

The epilogue also makes the important point that time marches forever forward: what is a good study today may be rendered obsolete tomorrow. And future breakthroughs will—not may—bring hope to present hopelessness. In late 2020, the TTTS and sIUGR outcomes are better than they were even five years ago, and with the election of a woman, Kamala Harris, to the vice presidency, perhaps American politics too will be more favorable for women's health. Writing now, I cannot know the contours of the next decade's scientific and political landscape. I therefore wish you the very best of luck, which made all the difference for me.

Challenging Pregnancy

Introduction

Antiabortion politics weren't responsible for my smaller twin coding in the NICU. It was why my twins and I were in intensive care in the first place. The twins' blood vessels had conjoined and had interwoven their fates and mine, but the red line of abortion divided us from the doctors who could have helped us, the procedures those doctors could have used, and the information available to me. In a contest of politics against science, politics won, at our expense and at the public's cost.

Americans vote according to their beliefs about abortion. For those who would ban it, abortion is the single issue that determines the candidate they support, even if the voter disagrees with the candidate on other important matters. But by supporting politicians who would prohibit all abortions at all costs and in all circumstances, antichoice Americans do themselves a great disservice: they drain the pool of physicians with the knowledge, skills, experience, and techniques to preserve a wanted pregnancy. When she is in need and her pregnancy has been struck with a bolt from the blue, the antiabortion voter will face the consequences of her single-issue ballot. No one will be left to save her.

As a lawyer specializing in reproductive rights advocacy, I intended to help someone else navigate the fraught politics of abortion. I presumed we Americans would eventually figure out our issues around reproductive choice, so that anyone I could help would live elsewhere, a place not as enlightened on human rights or as well resourced on healthcare as the United States. For someone less educated than I and somewhere poorer than here. That's where I could make a difference with my fancy degrees and forceful arguments demanding justice for pregnant women or newborn babies.

I certainly wasn't planning on advocating for myself. But I got pregnant, and my pregnancy was a disaster. How to help was beyond the expertise of most doctors, for they had not been educated about safely intervening to save a high-risk pregnancy. The few doctors knowledgeable about my condition were barred from assisting me by political obstacles, couched as technical or regulatory restrictions. I had to troll the internet late at night, unearthing medical articles from MedLine and the *Journal of the American Medical Association* (*JAMA*), doing reverse searches on the authors' names, tracing their professional histories until I could find where they currently worked. Then I would send pleading emails describing my condition and asking for a consultation, a phone call, an appointment, anything.

When the doctors where I lived in Washington, DC, didn't know what to do, I found a doctor in Baltimore. He disappeared for a while but reappeared when he took a job at another university. When his university hospital blocked him from assisting me further, I found still other doctors in Houston, Hollywood, and Miami. I had friends in LA, so I'd go to Hollywood! But Hollywood was a transcontinental flight away; how would I get to weekly prenatal appointments? Houston it was. I had no housing in Houston; Miami it would be. The doctor in Miami resigned from his hospital employer and moved to Belgium. Brussels is just seven hours across the Atlantic, and I could learn French. The outcomes from European studies, however, were not as encouraging as the American ones. Maybe it would be better if I stayed stateside?

I booked airline tickets, which I constantly changed. I exhausted the goodwill of friends and relatives, asking them to host me while I was in town, only to cancel my trips. I tried to remember my biostatistics classes from grad school—what was the odds ratio on that latest study? Was it better or worse than that other paper? What did it mean for me?

A pregnancy is only forty weeks—fewer if the birth is premature. My time to advocate and to analyze soon ran out. My babies came, regardless of my readiness for them and their readiness to be born. Some years later, I can report: we got lucky, we persevered, and we lived. That luck was a grace note, unearned, not merit based, not bought by education or wealth, though influenced by those factors. It was privileged by race and location. My babies and I didn't deserve this luck, no more so than a woman in an impoverished setting deserves her almost undoubtedly unlucky fate.

A pregnancy's outcome shouldn't depend on luck. My goal in writing this book is to explore and personalize the barriers to reproductive and maternal healthcare. More so than any other issue, abortion is the partition of American politics, the separator of red from blue.[1] Republican voters loyal to their party pledge to outlaw abortion, while Democrats vote to preserve women's ability to choose whether to continue a pregnancy. In *Challenging Pregnancy*, I argue that allowing doctors and patients to control decision-making around reproduction may safeguard the lives of those who are not seeking an abortion but who require cutting-edge care for an unanticipated and difficult pregnancy. The cost of outlawing or restricting abortion was almost three lives: my own and the twins'.

Throughout my pregnancy, I sought only my own and my family's survival and well-being, with my priorities in that order. It took all my education, experience, and privilege to try to obtain the care I required. At the eleventh hour, though, antiabortion politics and stigma served to vitiate those advantages. That could have killed us all.

Chapter One

Blighted Ovum

My husband's vision of growing old peacefully with his cat had been drastically disrupted, as had his plans for an early retirement. Ten years my senior, my spouse was struggling with the radical life changes brought by his late-life agreement to marry and to conceive a single child. We would have no more. I was content to nurse my one-year-old baby, who I hoped would soon learn to sleep through the night. And I needed to reclaim a career that had stalled with my first pregnancy's maternity leave and my breast milk–pumping breaks in a grimy, windowless basement closet my male colleagues used for phone calls to their mistresses.

My favorite boss, a blunt-spoken Dutch economist with bright red lipstick and dozens of silver wrist bangles, insisted that I rethink my views. We both worked on civil rights policies at a public health organization, but she gave short shrift to my feminist opposition to marriage and children. She also took full credit for having converted me, after years of badgering, from a swinging single to a married mother-of-one. Now, she applied her forthright approach to convincing me to have more children. I was unmoved by her demographic argument about the need to have 2.1 children as replacement population for my spouse and me. Then, she tried a different tack.

As we stood in line at the coffee cart outside our office, my boss squinted into the sun to pretend she wasn't crying and said hoarsely, "You must have another child, in case anything happens to the first." When he was thirteen, her son was struck by a car while skateboarding next to their house. He was comatose for two and a half years. Then, after aspirating on his own vomit, he died. If she hadn't had other children, she would have laid down and died as well. But her two daughters' needs forced her to push past her grief and continue to live.

My boss's latest argument was most persuasive and utterly heartbreaking. I prevailed upon my spouse for one more child, a spare to the heir. He agreed begrudgingly. Only one, at his insistence. He soon would turn fifty. In his view at half a century, the only diapers anyone should change were one's own. After this one single extra backup child, the baby-making factory would be closed, permanently. We would hire a nanny for the children, I'd go back to work, and having already achieved success in his career and being closer to retirement, he would be the primary child caretaker.

The pregnancy itself was easily accomplished. It took only three, well-timed tries for the home pregnancy test to come back positive. I kept that news to myself for ten weeks. When he found out about the pregnancy, true to his word, my husband never again put himself in a situation to conceive another child. The baby factory was closed, its workers laid off. Already, I could tell that our agreement of dividing child and home responsibilities between ourselves would never work.

But I didn't look or feel pregnant, and, according to the six-week ultrasound before Christmas, I wasn't pregnant. There was something in my uterus, a white, ghostly dot on the black ultrasound screen, but it was abnormal. They called it a "blighted ovum," which had implanted itself into the uterine wall but would never develop into a fetus, for a fertilized egg does not a pregnancy make. The egg could be of poor quality or the sperm that fertilized it chromosomally deficient. My body, sensing our failures and resulting aberrations, had stopped the pregnancy.[1] The gestational sac that should contain an embryo instead was an empty, crumpled sock, devoid of any developing life.

The headless horsemen of reproduction, blighted ova must be removed from the uterus; otherwise, they can cause hormonal and uterine problems for the woman they inhabit. Depending on the size of the ovum, various procedures could be used to expel it if it refused to be rousted on its own. A dilation and curettage (D&C) was prescribed as my remedy.

A D&C is a standard gynecological procedure used to remove any tissue that is in the uterus but shouldn't be: polyps, tumors, and, yes, whatever remains after a miscarriage, including a blighted ovum. Excess, useless tissue cannot stay inside the uterus or infection could result. From local infection, a blood infection or sepsis will spread wherever the blood flows and could be fatal. All the while, the pregnancy hormones will play on, tricked by the ovum into believing the body is pregnant, when it is, in fact, not.

Uteruses themselves are problematic organs. They are prone to tissue overgrowth, to infection, to bleeding. Without adequate gynecological care, having a uterus can kill you; every year, approximately 295,000 women die because of infections, hemorrhage, or hypertension related to pregnancy (including miscarriage, abortion, and postpartum conditions).[2] Most of these deaths are preventable if a woman has timely access to a skilled medical provider with the right tools and medicines. But in rich countries, poorly managed miscarriages, lack of treatment for ectopic pregnancies and other gynecological disorders, and inadequate postabortion care are the most important causes of pregnancy-related death.[3]

Indeed, despite its wealth, healthcare system, and global dominance, the United States, where I live, can be a dangerous place for those, like me, with uteruses. Maternal mortality in the United States has increased steadily over the past thirty years, with 17.4 women dying for every 100,000 who had a live birth in 2018.[4] The maternal mortality ratio of the United States is the highest of the fourteen most developed countries in the world, and it is rising while maternal deaths decrease elsewhere.[5]

A reason—perhaps *the* reason—for the high rate of pregnancy-related sickness and death for Americans is our lack of access to reproductive, maternal, and postpartum healthcare. Access can be considered in terms of a healthcare service's physical availability, economic affordability, and cultural appropriateness for the population that needs it.[6] In the United States, many procedures and medications used in gynecological and obstetric practice are prohibited by federal regulation or the laws of certain states, for fear that these tools could be used to procure an abortion. These prohibitions place medical standards of care, those medications and services provided by the prudent physician,[7] beyond the physical access of 72.7 million US women of reproductive age.[8] The politics of American pregnancy are what makes US maternity care terrible and difficult to obtain.

Consider the D&C my gynecologist prescribed for me: D&Cs are exceedingly common and so necessary for uterine healthcare that they happen in a doctor's office and take only five minutes. But the D&C procedure is invasive and requires a skilled practitioner because D&Cs can use sharp implements, and a poorly done D&C could perforate the uterus.[9] A D&C done in a gynecologist's office usually involves a paracervical block—this is a procedure that uses lidocaine injected adjacent to the cervix to numb those receptors. Some doctors sedate their patients using general anesthesia given intravenously. This lessens the patient's pain and anxiety over the procedure but requires special staff to administer, adding to the cost and length of the D&C. Doctors also may prescribe the patient medicine to open or "soften" her cervix. Then the woman lies on an examining table, her feet in stirrups, while the doctor inserts cervical dilators, long metal rods in increasing diameter, through her vagina into her cervix to dilate it. With the cervix open, the doctor then has access to the woman's uterus, which the doctor scrapes with a curette, a long, sharp spoon used to scoop out the uterine contents. Once the numbing agent wears off, the woman's cramps and vaginal bleeding will last for a few days.

My doctor could have scheduled me for a different procedure, a dilation and evacuation, the D&E, which is another way gynecologists remove tissue from uteruses when a less invasive surgical procedure is advised.[10] Mississippi, Nebraska, and West Virginia, however, had made D&E illegal in certain circumstances, and eight other states have attempted to do so.[11] Where D&E are proscribed, doctors have to perform D&Cs instead, even if these are not the ideal procedure for the patient.

Prohibition of medical procedures also means doctors are not trained to do them skillfully. Many ob/gyn residency training programs do not show doctors how to perform D&E procedures safely. Even beyond termination of pregnancy, there are always situations where a D&E is the better procedure. For a patient with a previable pregnancy who is hemorrhaging from an accident or trauma or from placenta previa, a doctor prohibited from doing a D&E would have to make a very large cut in the uterus to stop the bleeding. The patient would then be required to deliver by caesarean section in the future, presaging potential complications. A D&E done through the cervix only would be a safer procedure if a trained provider correctly used the right equipment.

Twenty-one states outlaw dilation and extraction (D&X) for pregnancy terminations.[12] D&X is a more complex surgery for patients who are miscarrying, to seek an autopsy of fetal remains, or to reduce potential trauma to the uterus from the introduction of sharp instruments during an abortion. It is exceedingly rare that a doctor would abort a pregnancy using a D&X. Because of state prohibitions on when D&X might be used, many medical students are not trained to perform D&X.[13] As a result, a cadre of doctors is leaving medical schools without the necessary skills or knowledge to resolve miscarriages.

Neither can American women easily obtain medications that are typically used in gynecological practice worldwide. The US Food and Drug Administration (FDA) has been "studying" the use of misoprostol for at least five years, but the agency has not approved this drug's use in gynecology.[14] Misoprostol is a drug developed to treat stomach ulcers, but it can be employed in other ways as well. Both the World Health Organization (WHO)[15] and the American College of Obstetricians and Gynecologists (ACOG)[16] recommend misoprostol to soften the cervix and to control blood loss in uterine surgery and childbirth. The FDA does not condone misoprostol for these purposes, warning of "serious side effects" from the medication's use. When American doctors use it, they must do so "off-label" or outside its approved purposes. Instead, the cervical ripening agent approved for labor induction in the United States for D&Cs is dinoprostone.

Why is the US government opposed to misoprostol, which is less expensive and more widely available than dinoprostone? The likely culprit for the barrier to Americans' access to this gynecological standard therapy is American antiabortion politics. In addition to using misoprostol to treat stomach ulcers, control blood sugar for those with Cushing's syndrome, and stanch hemorrhaging in labor and delivery, women throughout the world discreetly use misoprostol in combination with mifepristone (also known as RU-486) to terminate pregnancies.[17] In other countries, even those with restrictive abortion laws, these medicines are available over the counter and without prescription, permitting women to abort early pregnancies at home, according to their own will, and without the knowledge of government authorities or other people.

Until recently, American women like me could obtain misoprostol and mifepristone through the mail. Those in locations with limited access to doctors and reproductive healthcare providers, especially people living in rural or conservative states, placed internet orders with foreign doctors or pharmacies, who would mail the drugs directly to the patient. But this jig is up. In 2019, the FDA foreclosed mail-order access to both mifepristone and misoprostol.[18]

FDA's ever-increasing restrictions on medical abortion access are furthered through its Risk Evaluation and Mitigation Strategy (REMS) for the mifepristone. The FDA imposes a REMS on drugs that, ostensibly, could do more

harm than good if not regulated. Certain drugs, such as thalidomide, responsible for birth defects in the 1960s; isotretinoin, also linked to birth defects;
and fentanyl, abused in today's opioid crisis, have real health benefits but pose
significant dangers. A REMS is a regulatory attempt to control a drug's risks
so that its benefits are superior to its detriments.

The REMS for mifepristone includes the requirement that women seeking the drug must travel to obtain it in person at a doctor's office or hospital. Mifepristone cannot be dispensed like any other drug at a freestanding
pharmacy. Medical providers seeking to dispense mifepristone must serve as
their own pharmacy and keep a stock of the medication on hand. Providers may not write a prescription so that patients could obtain the drug at a
more convenient location—or without first making an appointment with a
doctor qualified to dispense mifepristone and with available stock. Finally,
before dispensing mifepristone, medical providers must obtain from each person intending to use the drug a signed patient agreement form, similar to the
iPLEDGE agreement for acne sufferers prescribed isotretinoin. In the agreement, the patient confirms that she is terminating a pregnancy, that she knows
the supposedly deleterious effects of taking mifepristone, and that she pledges
to assume these risks herself. She promises to take the drug only in accordance
with the law and the prescriber's instructions. In short, she absolves her doctor
of legal liability for her pregnancy termination and vows not to sue.

From the stringency of the restrictions applied to them, one might conclude that misoprostol and mifepristone are very dangerous drugs. But when
used in even higher dosages to treat ulcers or the side effects of Cushing's
syndrome, misoprostol is not subject to a REMS because few adverse effects
are associated with the drug's use. Fewer than one quarter of a percent of patients experience a serious medical complication from using mifepristone with
misoprostol to end a pregnancy.[19]

The biggest risks of mifepristone and misoprostol are not health-related at
all; they are political and calculated to restrict medical abortions.[20] The barriers to both drugs are not based on the drugs' public health harm. Instead, a
typical risk-benefit calculation is absent for these medications. If a medicine's
benefits far outweigh its risks, US regulatory authorities make that medication available to the public with, perhaps, labeling that describes whatever
risks the medication poses. Despite the ample evidence that both mifepristone

and misoprostol, when used individually and in combination, help the patient, with very few adverse outcomes, both doctors and patients must jump through several regulatory hoops to obtain these medications. Limiting access to both medicines places a barrier to women's self-management of abortion and miscarriage and to gynecologists' use of the misoprostol to support surgery and birth. These medicines are readily available outside the United States. But once again, as with D&Es and other gynecological procedures and medications, the standard of care is not available to Americans.

The only silver lining to COVID-19 is that the pandemic improved one aspect of reproductive healthcare access, even if temporarily, in the United States. In July 2020, a federal judge in Maryland suspended the FDA's longstanding restrictions on mifepristone used in combination with misoprostol to manage miscarriages or abortions at home.[21] Ruling that FDA's requirement of in-person doctors' visits during an infectious disease pandemic imposed a substantial obstacle to constitutionally protected abortion care, the court decreed that patients may receive both mifepristone and misoprostol from their doctors through the mail.[22] The judge's order applied nationwide and was to remain in effect until at least thirty days after the end of the US government's declared coronavirus public health emergency.

The district court poked a bear in the form of President Donald Trump, whose 2020 reelection platform mixed misogyny with COVID denials and contempt for public health and judicial norms. In October 2020, the Supreme Court ordered the District Court of Maryland to consider whether the pandemic had waned such that the FDA's motion to dissolve, modify, or stay the injunction could be granted.[23] The Trump administration argued to the Supreme Court that COVID infections were on the downswing, meaning patients had nothing to fear in waiting in doctors' offices and hospitals to retrieve their abortion medications.[24] Then, immediately before the election and in a ceremony that became a COVID superspreader, the president rushed through the Senate confirmation of a new Supreme Court justice, Amy Coney Barrett, an avowed opponent to reproductive rights and abortion.[25]

The federal district court refused to be cowed by the president and his Supreme Court. In December, it upheld its suspension of in-person requirements for those seeking medical abortions, citing the rapidly worsening COVID infection and death rates throughout the United States.[26] Zealous to curtail reproductive rights one final time, the Trump FDA audaciously bypassed the next level of appellate courts and directly petitioned the Supreme Court to overturn the district court's ruling. On January 12, 2021, a mere eight days before the end of President Trump's term, Justice Barrett made her mark. Ruling that courts could not substitute their evaluations of the effect of the pandemic for those of the public health experts at the FDA, the Supreme Court reinstated the requirement that those desiring to end their pregnancies must personally pick up their medications.[27]

The COVID crisis years of 2020 and 2021 made plain the difficulty all Americans have in accessing healthcare adequate to protect us against infectious diseases and all other medical needs. Antiabortion politics only exacerbates these difficulties, requiring patients to appear in a doctor's office for gynecological and obstetric care, when most other medical consultations could be handled by Zoom. Such was also the case in 2015, when I discovered I was a bearer of uterine blight. I was at the mercy of whoever could treat me with whatever tools available, regardless of whether the implements and procedures used were the state-of-the-art or just whatever politicians permitted for American women.

This state of affairs was disappointing but not soul crushing, and I was then too naïve to know that I could or should demand better. Because conception and pregnancy are so intensely personal, neither did I consider the public health or political ramifications of my situation, my professional experience as a reproductive health advocate notwithstanding. Any larger lessons I could have learned from needing to seek a quasi-pregnancy termination were utterly lost on me—at least, at first. I would get my D&C and would try again to conceive.

Given that I wasn't pregnant, there was no need to take the precautions of pregnancy. I enjoyed Christmas with my toddler and ate soft cheese and sushi in abundance. At midnight on January 1, I toasted the New Year with champagne. I looked into restarting my trapeze lessons and contemplated scuba diving over spring break. I told no one, including my spouse, about another potential pregnancy or its impending loss. Better to avoid causing excitement where there was none and to avert awkward or difficult conversations.

I presented myself at the gynecologist's a week after the New Year to remove the blighted ovum. Before the planned D&C, another ultrasound was done, just to be certain of the problem and its location. Scanning the depths of my uterus, my doctor gasped and said, "Oh! There's been a mistake. One was hidden behind the other. You're having twins."

I sat straight up, ultrasound gel running off my groin and said, "What the fuck do you mean?"

The doctor said, "I beg your pardon." I responded, "I beg yours."

I later sent my gynecologist an apology email. She was very gracious and said it was not the first time an angry patient lobbed an F-bomb on her. She reports swearing and provider-directed fury are common patient reactions to notification of a twin pregnancy. Because she subsequently did not drop me as a patient, I hereby dedicate this book to her.

Leaving my gynecologist, I staggered down the street and over a few blocks to my husband's office building to deliver the shocking news that I was pregnant twice over. I burst into his lobby, a never-before occurrence, to discover the entire staff, from partners to secretaries, staring at me from an adjacent, glassed-in conference room. I had walked directly into an ongoing all-hands meeting. My spouse, who had not expected my abrupt arrival, excused himself to figure out to what he owed the honor of my appearance. In his private office, he went white with shock on receiving the news and crumpled onto a couch. Once he recovered his capacity for speech, he informed me raising twins would be impossible at his age. I had gotten myself into this mess, and it remained my problem to resolve.

Chapter Two

"Freaks of Nature"

I n the United States, twin births per year doubled from around 70,000 in 1980 to 140,000 in 2010. Now, "multiples" of twins, triplets, and quadruplets represent 3 percent of all live births, with twins the vast majority. Most of the increase in the births of multiple babies is attributed to older women getting pregnant. As a woman's age advances, her hormonal levels rise, causing her to release more eggs per menstrual cycle.[1] If more than one egg is fertilized, one, two, or more zygotes, cell packets, may form. If all goes well and if considerable odds are overcome, in a bit over nine months, more than one baby will be born.

Statistics on the increasing age of mothers forecast a coming tidal wave of twins. Recently, for the first time in history, US women in their thirties gave birth more often than women in their twenties.[2] For teenaged moms, twin births happen only sixteen times per thousand live births, but there will be seventy sets of multiples in every group of thousand live births for mothers over forty years old. If the most common age of a woman pregnant with twins is thirty-nine and there is a baby boom in the birthrate for women aged thirty-five to forty-four,[3] the demographic trend is clear: there is a twin boom for older moms as well.

Those booming twins are all fraternal and not identical. They have been created from wholly separate eggs and different sperm, resulting in two separate zygotes, which grow to be distinct, different-looking children. Fraternal twins' genetic relationship is like that of any other siblings; these twins can be opposite sexes, a boy and a girl. Their similarity is merely that they have shared a womb and have the same birthday.

A number of factors can lead to conceiving nonidentical twins. In addition to increased maternal age, use of assisted reproductive technologies (ART), often by older mothers, is associated with the increase in fraternal twins. Americans' reliance on in vitro fertilization (IVF), an ART form, is ever increasing, from 1.6 percent of all 2013 births to 2.15 percent of all live births in 2018.[4] Now in the United States, almost half of the children born through IVF are from a pregnancy of twins, triplets, or more.[5]

Being Afro-descendent rather than Caucasian makes a woman more likely to have fraternal twins—no one knows why. Fraternal twins also run in families, so if you are a nonidentical twin, you are more likely to conceive nonidentical twins. And, proving that nature has a twisted sense of humor, if a mother already has had fraternal twins, her next pregnancy is more likely to be another set of nonidentical twins.

What has not changed at all over three decades is the number of identical twins. Identical twins are and will forever be rare. If 3 percent of births are now multiples, only 3 percent of that 3 percent are identical twins. The conception of identical twins is unrelated to a woman's age, race, use of reproductive technologies,[6] or genetics. The peak incidence of fraternal twins is 1.4 percent for women aged forty; however, the incidence of identical twins for women of any age is around a third of a percent.

Identical twins are monozygotic, or formed from the same egg and sperm. The resulting single zygote splits early in its development, creating two separate cell groupings that contain the same genetic material from one egg and one sperm. These twins are nature's clones and are always the same sex.

A fight with my husband over having twins was itself premature because the ultrasound results were not encouraging. Two nine-week-old, implanted embryos should have been clearly visible and about the same size. Something seemed very wrong with one of the embryos—it was much smaller than the other and could hardly be detected, which is why, on the first ultrasound, it wasn't seen at all. At this stage of the pregnancy, if my body were to expel one of the embryos, I would miscarry both.

How to clean up the mess fell on my shoulders alone. My husband was not at all happy about this turn of events. Instead of thinking about how to proceed, he preferred instead to schedule a ski trip getaway for the beginning of February. I had to unearth my buried public health research skills.

Maternal and infant health issues had propelled me into public health. My sixteenth birthday was spent in Bolivia, volunteering with the poorest women

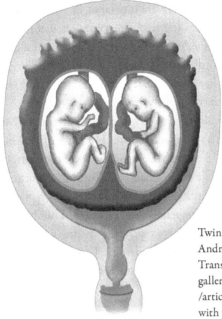

Twin fetuses. From Lisa M. Moore and Andres Manuel Biaggi, "Twin-to-Twin Transfusion Syndrome," April 2, 2020, media gallery 2, https://emedicine.medscape.com /article/271752-overview. Image reproduced with permission from Medscape Drugs & Diseases (www.emedicine.medscape.com).

and children in the Western Hemisphere. My aunt and uncle lived in La Paz, but my aunt had been evacuated from that high-altitude location because of her own pregnancy complications. I found her copy of *Our Bodies, Ourselves* stashed in the bathroom. Reading that book was a revelation. Although my conservative upbringing had involved protesting with my family outside of abortion clinics, *Our Bodies, Ourselves* educated me about the ease with which women could fall pregnant, the life-threatening consequences of pregnancy, and women's desperation to terminate pregnancies that threatened their health or their aspirations. There would be no more abortion clinic protests for me; I would be on the side of women.

At nineteen, I helped a teenaged migrant farmworker give birth in North Carolina. She was a year younger than I and had been abandoned by the older boyfriend who brought her across the US border from Mexico. When I met her at the rural health clinic where I was assigned that summer, she was nine months pregnant and due at any second. The clinic supervisor told me to be on call to drive the girl to the hospital when she went into labor. She also handed me a VHS tape of midwifery techniques and told me to watch it, just in case we didn't make it to the hospital in time. We arrived in time for a hospitalized birth, after breaking land-speed records over the twenty-mile trip. But the girl had no family or friends to attend her birth. She (and the hospital's staff) let me apply my video learning to catch the baby as she emerged.

By twenty, I was a Peace Corps volunteer in Kyrgyzstan, Central Asia. My assignment was to teach English in a village school, and I found it distressing that some of my best students would disappear overnight, never to return to class. The other girls told me their classmates had been "stolen." A form of forced marriage, bride stealing is a harmful, traditional practice in which a girl is kidnapped, raped, and often impregnated at an early age.[7] I hitchhiked to the capital and talked the UNICEF country representative into permitting me to develop a national girls' rights program based on the Convention on the Rights of the Child. For good measure, I also became certified as a lactation consultant and set up mothers' and doctors' breastfeeding groups throughout the country.

My short life's experiences with women's reproductive health made me want to be a doctor, but poor university grades in physics made medical school admission unlikely. So, from Central Asia, I applied to join law and public health graduate programs. If I couldn't help individual women and girls with their pregnancies, I could change the system to improve the conditions of pregnancy for everyone. Eventually, I gained admission to a very good law school, Georgetown, and the world's best public health school, Johns Hopkins.

After graduation, I took a succession of health policy and advocacy jobs. These involved writing drafts of legislation on reproductive health and lobbying governmental officials to pass these drafts—or to fund the programs they would support. On a typical day, I would meet with staff of members of the US Congress and patiently explain the purpose of male or female condoms. I learned to smile beatifically when legislators told me that unwanted pregnancies would be resolved by having a "strong male presence" in the household. I joined the board of directors of a maternal and infant health organization in Malawi, where unassisted childbirths are as ubiquitous as postpartum deaths of women and infants. A decade passed in which I never once used biostatistics to determine the reliability of research or the applicability of a study's conclusion to a wider population. Until now, during my own pregnancy. Apparently, now I was gestating zombie twins, which were neither fully alive nor completely dead.

I investigated the possibility of a selective reduction, terminating one embryo to save the other. Selective reduction is the polite term for a socially acceptable abortion because of the risks involved in carrying multiple fetuses to term. Many pregnancies of three or more embryos are reduced, usually to twins.[8] The American College of Obstetricians and Gynecologists (ACOG) reports that "infants born after a multifetal pregnancy are at increased risk of prematurity, cerebral palsy, learning disabilities, slow language development, behavioral difficulties, chronic lung disease, developmental delay, and death."[9] Reducing the pregnancy by one or more fetuses decreases the risk of miscarriage of the entire pregnancy or of stillbirth of the babies. The most dramatic benefits from selective reductions are for reductions of pregnancies with three or more fetuses.[10] ACOG instructs that all patients pregnant with multiples should be counseled about the risks of higher order pregnancies. Fewer babies from one pregnancy are safer, both for the mother and for the remaining fetuses.[11] All options, including reduction, should be offered to the patient, with the doctor ultimately respecting the patient's autonomy to determine the course of the pregnancy.

Selective reductions (and sensible assisted reproduction practices, which are only suggestions in the United States but are legally mandated elsewhere) are why there has been only one Octomom, a woman who had eight babies in one go. After her fertility doctor implanted a stunning twelve embryos in her uterus, Nadya Suleman's obstetricians strongly encouraged her to reduce her pregnancy.[12] She refused and instead gave birth to premature octuplets in 2009, resulting in extended hospitalizations for her and the babies. Other women in Ms. Suleman's position have followed their doctors' advice and reduced their fetuses to a safer, more manageable number. Surely, I thought, if selective reductions could be done for the world's Octomoms, they could be done for women carrying two embryos. I discovered, though, that selective reductions for twins are highly controversial and seldom offered, ACOG's guidance notwithstanding.[13] A twin pregnancy is a risky proposition for the mother and babies, but most doctors do not deem these risks significant enough to warrant a reduction of two fetuses to one.

What are these risks? Twins' risk of cerebral palsy is four times higher than for a single baby, and twins are seven times more likely to die before their first birthday. This is because most twins are born premature and at low birth weights. Although twins are only 3 percent of all live births, they are 17 percent of preterm births before 37 weeks of gestation. And they are 23 percent of all very preterm births before 32 gestational weeks. On average, twins are born at only 35 weeks. Because they haven't spent enough time growing inside their mothers, most newborn twins are under 2,500 grams, or 5.5 pounds. Over 10 percent of twins weigh fewer than 1,500 grams, 3.3 pounds, at birth.

Twins are also dangerous for those carrying them. Women pregnant with twins have an almost four times greater risk for preeclampsia—when soaring high blood pressure can lead to stroke—than women pregnant with a singleton. The risk for gestational diabetes, which is related to developing diabetes later in life, is two times as great. More than a quarter of twin pregnancies are in danger of ending in miscarriage, often leading to hemorrhaging and blood loss. The relative risk for blood clots during pregnancy and after birth is three times and twice as high, respectively, as for women pregnant with one fetus. And, compared with the almost 2 percent of singleton mothers who, like Great Britain's Duchess Kate, suffer hyperemesis, or debilitating nausea and vomiting during pregnancy, more than 5 percent of twin mothers are afflicted with this condition.

Twins also are terribly expensive, both financially and emotionally. Compared to a pregnancy of a single baby, medical costs are quadrupled for a twin pregnancy. In 2005, eons ago, a hospitalized birth averaged $9,800 for a singleton but cost $38,000 for twins.[14] (Costs have increased since then.) A stay in the neonatal intensive care unit (NICU), costs $3,500 per baby per day; many twins are in the NICU for weeks.[15] Parents of twins report severe stress, higher rates of depression, and a compromised quality of life. Child abuse is more common in families raising twins, and twin parents are more likely to divorce.[16]

I placed discreet phone calls to maternal and fetal medicine specialists in the DC area, asking about reducing twin fetuses to a singleton. The response was always a shocked silence followed by an emphatic denial that such a procedure could be done. No, a referral could not be made to a doctor who would be willing to reduce twins. No one knew any doctor engaged in such a practice.

My internet searches led me to one doctor in New York City who would selectively reduce *fraternal* twin pregnancies from two embryos to one. That small detail turned out to be consequential. I called to make an appointment with the doctor and arranged to meet my husband on the ski trip the day following the appointment. My husband and child would fly out West, and I would catch up with them a day later. My spouse, who, by then had completely removed himself mentally from any worries about the pregnancy, urged me not to tarry in NYC. He complained that it would be difficult and stressful to take care of a toddler all by himself. But more to the point, we'd miss valuable time on the slopes.

Hanging up the phone, I left for work and exited the metro smack into the annual, late January antiabortion protest commemorating the *Roe v. Wade* decision. Teenagers, likely far too young to have had sex, much less children of their own, surged around me. Waving giant, six-foot-tall placards displaying bloody fetal parts, they chanted, "We are abortion survivors." I was both annoyed by the fallacy of their chant—abortions are of nonviable fetuses, so no living human could have survived an abortion, much less a crowd of them gathered at the same metro stop—and gutted by their crappy timing and targeting of me. How could they have known what I was experiencing and contemplating? Years earlier, though, I could have been one of them, protesting abortions I could not understand. They were glib, and so was I. Now, I said to one of the teens, "May you never have to experience a wanted but impossible pregnancy."

My gynecologist was worried about whatever the ultrasounds were saying, but she also was overbooked. My next appointment would not be until my twelfth week of gestation, which would be too far along for a selective reduction or easy termination of the entire pregnancy. I sought an appointment with a specialty, high-risk obstetrician, who could explain what was happening with the two embryos: was there hope for both, or should I reduce the pregnancy? Finally, a high-risk OB agreed to see me when I was at 10.5 weeks, and five days before my selective reduction appointment in NYC.

Several radiology techs and a team of doctors stood around me to view the ultrasound projected on a screen across the room. The image was of a goldfish and a tadpole surrounded by bubbles. The bubble around the tadpole was conspicuously smaller than that around the goldfish, and both bubbles were lassoed together. The radiologist moved the cursor on the computer screen over the neck area of one fetus and measured a pocket of fluid, the nuchal translucency: 3.2 millimeters. High, not normal. A potential sign of cardiovascular problems. After some hemming and hawing, the doctors rendered their verdict: twin-to-twin transfusion syndrome, which occurs only with identical twins.

Although many things—the age and race of the mother, genetics, use of assisted reproduction methods—can lead to fraternal twins, identical twins are "freaks of nature." No one knows why they occur, but everyone agrees that pregnancies with identical twins are particularly problematic. The problems inherent to identical twins are portended by the intrauterine sacs in which they develop. Within a woman's uterus, a fetus is enclosed within a bag of waters, the amniotic sac, which is surrounded by an internal membrane, the amnion. The amniotic sac's external membrane is called the chorion. The placenta feeds the fetus and excretes its wastes. "The placenta" is also the answer to the famous Trivial Pursuit question, "What is the only organ that is grown, regrown, and expelled by the body?" An umbilical cord connects the placenta to the fetus.

Because fraternal twins originate from distinct eggs and sperm, which form separate zygotes that grow into individual embryos, these fetuses develop in separate amniotic sacs with separate chorions. There are "di," or two, of each: two zygotes, two embryos, two fetuses, two amnions, two chorions. The mother grows two placentas, one to nourish each twin. The shorthand for these dichorionic/diamniotic twins is di-di or DCDA.

In contrast to dizygotic fraternal twins, identical twins must share all they have from the very start. The identical twins are monozygotic, formed from the same single sperm and egg, which develop a single fertilized egg or zygote. Exactly when during its development the zygote splits to form two embryos determines how much the twins must share; the earlier the split, the greater the differentiation between the twins.[17] There are three possibilities. In exceedingly rare cases, the zygote cleaves, or splits, by the third day after fertilization, leading to the identical twins, each in its own amniotic sac with its own chorion.[18] Two amniotic sacs and two chorions mean these twin fetuses are called di-di, just like fraternal DCDA twins.

In the more typical case for identical twins, the zygote splits in half between four and eight days after fertilization. The twin embryos will form in separate amniotic sacs contained within the same outer membrane. Such twins have one (mono) chorion and two (di) sacs. They are designated as monochorionic/diamniotic or mono-di or MCDA.

Two percent of twins share a single amniotic sac with a single chorion resulting from zygotes that split even later than mono-di twins. Monochorionic/monoamniotic twins' zygotes cleave eight to twelve days after fertilization; too late to develop separate amniotic sacs. These twin fetuses gestate in a single amniotic sac with only one chorion. The nickname for these twins is mono-mono, or MCMA, indicating these twins are monochorionic and monoamniotic. With no bag or membrane to separate them, they share their amniotic fluids and risk entangled umbilical cords. If a zygote attempts to split after twelve days postfertilization, the zygote may not cleave completely in half. The resulting twins will be conjoined, their bodies stuck together at the structures that were developing where the zygote did not separate. Conjoined twins are, by definition, also mono-mono, sharing both the amniotic sac and chorion.

I had made the appointment with the NYC selective reduction doctor with the expectation that I was carrying fraternal twins. The suspicion that my twins were identical changed the story entirely. I called the doctor's office to confirm my appointment, and the surgical nurse told me firmly that identical twin pregnancies could not be reduced; only fraternal twins could. Because identical twins may develop in the same amniotic sac, to reduce one would be to abort the entire pregnancy. The doctor was a fetal surgeon and not an abortionist, a word the nurse pronounced with distaste. The nurse rang off from the call, canceling my appointment and saying, "Good luck to you." I would remain pregnant with two embryos. At least my husband's ski trip would not be inconvenienced by my New York detour.

(*Chapter Three*)

Dr. Google

Google has revolutionized the doctor-patient relationship in that, with a few mouse clicks, every patient can seek information on any condition. The problem is that most patients are ill-equipped to understand their consultation with Dr. Google, and discerning credible sources of information is challenging. If one is inclined to believe conspiracy theories and fake news, Google's algorithm will direct you to falsehoods and sensationalized articles.[1] These will lead down a rabbit hole, each linking to another discredited source, until your view of reality is wholly skewed and Google's artificial intelligence (AI) fully trained to deliver you poor quality information for your subsequent searches. But if the AI has pegged someone as typically searching out neutral and truthful material, exactly this will appear at the top of your search results. As you consume articles from recognized news organizations, medical journals, and vetted sources, again the AI learns your interests and requirements. The next time you search, the very sources you would likely read appear front and center, almost as if someone read your mind and knew what you were searching for. Of course, advertisers in Google know how to play this game. They can pay to have their source listed first in a Google search, thereby subverting your AI results with their financial or political motives.

Even if your Google search profile indicates you would be receptive to correct and honest information, reliability requires more than the information's not coming from a wackadoodle source with suspect motives for publishing it on the internet. The information should be written by someone with expertise in the issue reported; it should be gathered from a trial with a control; it should be peer-reviewed; and it should be published in an indexed journal. Searching within Google Scholar assists in assuring the information you receive has been published by experts and has been reviewed by the peers of those experts, who are also authorities in their fields. Most—but, maddeningly, not all—sources in Google Scholar are from "indexed journals," meaning that these sources are considered of high scientific quality.[2] Indexed journals are listed in compilations, such as MedLine and PubMed, that universities use in the conduct of their research and in their evaluation of professorial research for tenure decisions.

But one properly using Google Scholar to search for information about an issue is still deluged with hundreds or thousands of articles to digest. How is the layperson to sort the wheat from the chaff? Again, my public health degree paid off, as I had learned the difference between a retrospective cohort study and a case-controlled study.[3] The best, most reliable information is gathered from trials where the outcome of one intervention (say, surgery) in one group of people is compared against a group that did not receive the intervention. Participants in these two groups should be selected randomly, and if possible, no participants should know whether they have received the intervention or a placebo that would have no effect.

Contrasting with randomized, controlled trials are retrospective cohort studies, which have no real-time control group. Participants in these studies have all received an intervention and are later contacted by researchers to learn of the outcome of the intervention. Retrospective studies often may be the only ethical way to research a medical intervention or public health risk. To study the benefits of seatbelt use, for example, it would be wrong to ask a control group not to wear seatbelts, given the fatal consequences of foregoing this risk reduction measure. Yet in retrospective studies, participants' recollections may be affected by time or bias or may simply be incorrect. If there are too few participants in a retrospective study, the study's conclusions cannot be generalized to the general population, as the data from which conclusions could be drawn are insufficiently limited. Further, when researchers are unable to collect data from many of the original study participants because they have dropped out of the study or have otherwise not responded to the research questions, the study cannot provide an accurate snapshot of what outcome could accurately be tied to the issue examined.

Therefore, a search for information should seek the outcomes from the gold standard of public health research, a randomized, controlled trial. When no controlled study is available, the maxim of "bigger is better" applies to any retrospective study consulted. Study results should be derived from results from many participants, and few participants should have dropped out of the study or been lost to follow-up. And, as with analyzing the sources listed from any Google search, the financial and political motives of the study authors should be born in mind. Credible studies and researchers disclose any conflicts in the very first paragraph of the study.

The results of googling twin-to-twin transfusion (or transfer) syndrome are objectively terrifying, and even an evil social media bot could not exaggerate the grim outlook. A typical medical article reports, "Twin-to-twin transfusion syndrome (TTTS) is the most important cause of handicap and death in monochorionic twin pregnancies."[4] Untreated TTTS results in virtually certain death of at least one fetus, likely mental retardation of the surviving fetus, and potential hemorrhaging of the mother.

TTTS affects only 10 percent of monochorionic twins, those rare, 3 percent of embryos that share the same placenta but that have separate amniotic sacs and membranes. When fetuses share a placenta, there will always be blood vessels from each that connect on the surface of the chorion. These vascular anastomoses allow blood from one twin to flow to the other twin. TTTS results when the anastomoses are unbalanced, with preferential shunting from one twin to the other.[5] One twin is the unwitting donor, transfusing the recipient twin with its blood. The donor twin has less blood, so it has fewer nutrients, grows more slowly, and is much smaller. Without the water from blood, the dehydrated donor also cannot produce urine. In a condition called oligohydramnios, no urine also means no amniotic fluid for the donor because amniotic fluid is merely fetus pee. With no fluid to inflate its amniotic sac, the sac's membrane droops over the fetus, clinging to it and gluing the fetus to the placental wall. Severe oligohydramnios can also lead to lack of or poor lung development in the donor. Fetal lungs need to be bathed in amniotic fluid to develop properly. Being "glued" can lead to joint and musculoskeletal deformities as well.

The recipient twin suffers the ill effects of being pumped full of the donor's blood. The recipient's heart struggles to keep up with the extra blood and may develop incorrectly—or the fetus may have heart failure, causing his body to swell with extreme hypertension. More blood means more urine, and the recipient twin has polyhydramnios, urinating with such frequency and volume that its amniotic sac balloons with liquid. The pressure from the overinflated amniotic sac can cause the sac to break, leading to preterm birth before the fetuses are viable.

The blood vessel connection of the donor and recipient further intertwines their fates. If either fetus should die—the donor from dehydration or the recipient from a heart attack—the survivor's blood pressure will drop precipitously, causing a hemorrhage to the deceased fetus that usually will kill the survivor. Or the survivor may suffer extreme brain damage and physical disability when its twin perishes.

TTTS is staged from I to V according to features seen on ultrasound and first categorized by Dr. Ruben Quintero, a preeminent fetal surgeon.[6] In TTTS, no matter the stage, the recipient and donor fetuses have polyhydramnios and oligohydramnios, too much and too little amniotic fluid, respectively. To be considered oligohydramnios, the deepest vertical pocket (DVP) of amniotic fluid around the donor fetus must be fewer than two centimeters, representing only the fifth percentile for amniotic fluid measurements. What is polyhydramnios differs in the United States and in Europe. In the United States, a TTTS recipient fetus is surrounded by a fluid pocket that is at least eight centimeters, or greater than the ninety-fifth percentile for amniotic fluid depths.[7] In Europe generally, a cut off for polyhydramnios is, as in the United States, a DVP of more than eight centimeters before 20 weeks of gestation.[8] The Belgians, however, suggest diagnosing TTTS if, before 18 weeks, the recipient's DVP is greater than six centimeters.[9] After 20 weeks, the Europeans diagnose TTTS only when the recipient's DVP is more than ten centimeters deep.[10]

At Stage I, the donor twin's bladder is still visible in an ultrasound; this early TTTS is characterized primarily by the fluid discrepancy between the fetuses' amniotic sacs. At Stage II, the donor's bladder is no longer visible, having failed to fill because the fetus has stopped urinating. By Stage III, the twins have absent or reversed blood flow in the umbilical artery, reverse flow in the ductus venosus (a special passageway important for a fetus' blood circulation), or flickering on-off flow in the umbilical vein. Stage IV is characterized by hydrops, which is when fluid builds up not only in the amniotic sac but also in the recipient's tissues and organs, causing extreme swelling. At Stage V, one or both twins die in utero.

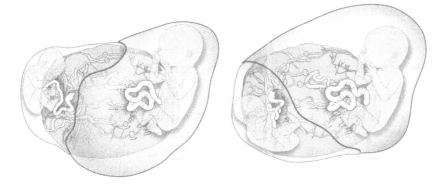

Donor twin stuck under amniotic membranes. From L. Van Der Veeken, I. Couck,
J. Van Der Merwe, L. De Catte, R. Devlieger, J. Deprest, and L. Lewi, "Laser for Twin-
to-Twin Transfusion Syndrome: A Guide for Endoscopic Surgeons," *Facts, Views and
Vision in Obstetrics and Gynecology* (September 2019): 197–205, 200, fig. 4, https://www
.ncbi.nlm.nih.gov/pmc/articles/PMC7020942/. Image reproduced with permission
from UZ Leuven (www.uzleuven.be).

Death of at least one twin is virtually certain if TTTS is not resolved. One
or both fetuses die in more than 80 percent of untreated TTTS cases. The
20 percent who survive are severely disabled, usually with mental retardation,
kidney, and cardiac defects. Without successful intervention, the outlook for
TTTS twins is "hopeless."[11] The mother carrying TTTS twins risks preterm
birth, blood clots, stroke, hemorrhaging, and the mental trauma of watching
her newborns perish moments after birth. Even with intervention, TTTS is
described as "devasting" and "a major challenge."[12]

High-risk obstetricians schedule their patient appointments two weeks
apart—just enough time to torture anxious parents. If I wanted answers, I had
to find them myself. I reactivated my subscriptions to PubMed and JSTOR,
two large databases of medical research. Then I started Boolean searches:
"twin-to-twin transfusion syndrome" or "TTTS" and "survival outcomes"
and "intervention" or "best practice" but not "maternal death."

After sorting for articles published only over the past two years, a few leads
popped up. These I scanned for the lead author's name and contact information. I started firing off emails, some of which bounced immediately. Each

bounce-back led to another Google search for the author's current location, usually at a university-affiliated hospital. Googling @universityname.edu gave me a few examples of email addresses for people at that university, which allowed me to try emailing the article authors again. In a typical email, I wrote:

Dear Dr. W

I have just read the 2010 article you coauthored in Ultrasound about selective reduction (SR) of monochorionic-diamniotic (mono-di) twins in complicated pregnancies. I wonder if you or a colleague are still performing these procedures. (I've also just emailed another co-author.)

I am just shy of 11 weeks pregnant with mono-di twins. Already, my high-risk ob, Dr. X, is concerned about twin-twin transfusion syndrome (TTTS). One of the fetuses is substantially larger than the other, and that large fetus also has a nuchal translucency measure of 3.2.

I asked about SR in mono di twins where one has a problem. Dr. X said this was not theoretically possible; and Dr. Y in NYC, whom I also consulted by telephone, concurred. I am told that I would have to terminate both fetuses.

Your article gave me some hope that SR may be an available option for mono-di twins. Would you please tell me if this is the case? If so, who might do these procedures and at what point in the pregnancy?

I am willing to travel to receive care, and I have very good health insurance.

Thank you for your time, and please excuse my bothering you.

Sincerely yours,

GG

Every fetal specialist I wrote returned my message. Each doctor explained that TTTS is no longer as hopeless as it once was, although the options for treatment are expensive, difficult, and experimental. Survival rates for the twins and the mother are better than they were even a decade ago. Doctors, however, do not agree about the best way to treat TTTS, especially TTTS at stages I and II, and which of the intervention choices leads to the most optimal outcome of two healthy, mentally and physically sound babies and a living mother.[13]

It turns out that selective reduction remains an option in TTTS, even though the fetuses are identical. How the pregnancy is reduced is different from standard selective reduction. For most selective reductions, potassium chloride is injected through the mother's uterus into the heart of a fetus. TTTS can be resolved through a procedure called cord coagulation, where a fetal surgeon uses a scope to enter the uterus with a laser to cauterize the umbilical cord of the sicker embryo. This cuts the blood supply to the fetus. If cord coagulation is done at sixteen weeks postfertilization, the sickest fetus will die and be absorbed by the placenta, allowing the healthier twin to continue to grow. Beyond the certainty that one twin will perish from cord coagulation, there are considerable risks to this TTTS treatment option. The amniotic sac may break when the fetoscope is inserted, resulting in the loss of both twins. The earlier the cord coagulation is performed, the greater the risk of membrane rupture. Or the operation may occur too late to save the larger twin or to ensure the survivor's health. The survivor's brain or heart may already have been damaged by the excess blood from the smaller twin.

Amnioreduction is another TTTS treatment alternative. This involves repetitively draining the engorged amniotic sac of the recipient twin. Guided by an ultrasound, the surgeon inserts a needle into the amniotic sac and removes up to a gallon of fluid. Because amnioreduction does not change the blood transfer from the donor to recipient twin, the procedure must be repeated every few weeks, as fluid will continue to build around the recipient. With each needle insertion, the surgeon risks breaking the amniotic sac and putting the mother in preterm labor. Only 60 percent of TTTS twins survive with amnioreduction, and 20 to 25 percent of survivors are brain damaged or disabled.[14]

The final alternative for TTTS is fetal laser surgery, but there are few doctors skilled and practiced with this intervention. Similar to cord coagulation, the surgeon inserts a laparoscope into the uterus. The scope has a camera, a fetoscope, which allows the doctor to identify the blood vessels connecting across the chorion membrane. The fetoscope has a second channel through which the surgeon passes a laser into the larger amniotic sac of the recipient twin. The laser is used to cauterize the connecting blood vessels, thereby separating the twins and stopping the blood transfusion from the donor to the recipient. Laser surgery is generally reserved for TTTS cases that have advanced beyond Quintero stage II.[15] The preferred surgical method is called the "Solomon technique," after the biblical king who proposed splitting a baby in half. Instead of undertaking a mission of searching and destroying each individual blood vessel that connects the fetuses, the surgeon draws a line with the laser from one side of the placenta. This technique slices and coagulates all possible anastomoses that lead from one fetus to the other, ensuring that no blood vessel is missed that may continue to permit the imbalance of blood between the twins.[16] Laser surgery thus treats the cause of TTTS. It also prevents brain and heart damage to the recipient if the donor twin dies and the recipient twin hemorrhages into the deceased fetus.

Fetal laser surgery is a high-wire balancing act. The damage could already be done, and the surgery can make the situation worse. The surgery can inadvertently kill one or both twins by disrupting their blood circulation and nutrient delivery or by breaking their amniotic sacs. It can cause the mother to give birth prematurely, long before the twins could survive. Or it could result in life with very poor quality. With the surgery, at least one twin survives 75 percent of the time, but around 9 percent of the survivors have "severe neurological illness": cerebral palsy, significant cognitive or motor delay, bilateral deafness, or complete blindness.[17] Surgery that does not completely separate the connecting placental blood vessels may not interrupt the ongoing blood transfusion of one fetus from the other. TTTS can recur or a related condition, twin anemia-polycythemia sequence (TAPS), may develop, increasing the risk of neurological damage to the twins.[18]

With an 80 percent certainty of death for the twins if I did nothing and a potential 75 percent survival rate from an intervention, it was clear that I should intervene—but how? I was not interested in creating life for life's sake; I wanted neurologically sound, healthy children who would have a decent quality of life. Web pages for hospitals throughout the United States repeat the same death and survival statistics for TTTS interventions. There are few current studies to back these statistics, however, and little information about the lives of children born after different TTTS interventions.

The ultimate goal of fetal therapy should be survival without neurodevelopmental impairment, but there remains medical debate about how to achieve that goal.[19] The seminal article about TTTS was written in 2000, but this article described the progression of the syndrome, not the long-term effects to its survivors.[20] At the time I was pregnant in 2015, a large European study examining the neurological and physical effects of TTTS was underway, but results were not released until 2016.[21] It was not until 2020, as I was writing this book, that results were anticipated from a randomized, controlled clinical study that compared the neonatal and infant health outcomes of fetal surgery versus doing nothing in a TTTS scenario that, ultimately, matched my own.[22]

Scanning my lists of coauthors of articles about TTTS, I located one specialist who had founded the fetal surgery practice at the University of Maryland and who was one of the pioneers in using intrauterine fetal surgery to resolve TTTS. But he seemed to have disappeared from UM. A few days later, he popped up again in a celebratory email from my alma mater—Johns Hopkins had poached him from Maryland to head Hopkins's new fetal surgery practice.

Having graduated from Hopkins's public health school, I knew the institution's firstname.lastname email address convention. I boldly wrote this lauded superstar doctor directly. I contemplated that no harm had ever come from asking a question and that no doctor would reject an offer to spend piles of money on his services. Further, email's impersonality would save me from any embarrassment I might feel asking for help. I should be no more concerned about writing a cutting-edge fetal researcher than I would be about contacting a contractor to mow the lawn or clean the gutters.

> Dear Dr. Z,
> I am 11 weeks pregnant with mono-di twins who likely have twin-twin transfusion syndrome (TTTS). My own research indicates that laser surgery may be an available option for mono-di twins. Would you please tell me if this is the case in the greater Washington-Baltimore area? If so, who might do these procedures and at what point in the pregnancy?
>
> Sincerely yours,
GG

The email left my fingertips at midnight. By 9:00 a.m., my telephone was ringing; it was Dr. Z. Could I drive to Baltimore right away? That same day? He was just setting up shop at Hopkins, but he would be happy to see me. He didn't really have an office yet, but he would borrow some space from the OB ward and meet me there. He might also bring some colleagues if that would be all right with me.

The high nuchal translucency results I received at my 10.5-week ultrasound could have indicated that at least one fetus had a chromosomal abnormality, such as Down syndrome. I opted for the earliest genetic test possible to determine whether the fetuses had any genetic defects that would convince me to end the pregnancy. Already, my husband and I doubted our ability to raise twins. There was no way we would be able to provide the life-long care necessary for a child severely compromised by a nontreatable condition. In fact, if genetic testing found problems with one twin, our future would be even more bleak. Because identical twins share a placenta and have the same genetic constitution, the testing results would foretell genetic diseases and problems for both twins. Two babies seemed impossible; two sick babies would be unbearable.

As with all things pregnancy, timing is everything. The earlier the abortion, the easier it is to find a doctor willing to terminate the pregnancy and the safer the abortion. In my area of the United States, abortions are not difficult to obtain in the first twelve weeks of pregnancy. After the first trimester, though, few locations and fewer doctors are available to terminate a pregnancy, even if the fetus is likely to have genetic malformations. More complicated still is when the woman lives in one of several states where the law dictates the first trimester of pregnancy as beginning with the woman's last menstrual period—two weeks before conception of that pregnancy. The trick is to find, schedule, and conduct a genetic test; receive the testing results; and then, if necessary, find, schedule, and receive an abortion while still in the jurisdiction's legally defined first trimester.

Chorionic villus sampling (CVS) can be done just after ten weeks of gestation. In CVS, a large hollow needle is used to puncture the woman's uterus and to remove a sample of fetal cells from the placenta. The cells are analyzed for a panoply of malformations, additions, or deletions in the fetus's chromosomes. The results are sent in a week. This quick turnaround allows women to schedule additional testing and to make pregnancy termination decisions still early in the pregnancy and, in most but not all states, before the end of the first trimester.

CVS is not without some risk, depending on the timing of the procedure and the skill and experience of the doctor performing it.[23] In 1 percent of cases, CVS causes a miscarriage.[24] Especially in CVSes conducted before eleven weeks of gestation, punching a small hole in the uterus can cause the woman's muscles to contract and expel her fetus. Or in CVSes before ten weeks, an inexperienced doctor might misread the ultrasound guiding the needle placement and accidentally send micro–blood clots to the fetus or disrupt blood flow sufficiently to cause the tiny fingers and toes to resorb and disappear.[25]

An alternative to CVS is amniocentesis, which poses a lower risk of miscarriage and birth defects but must be conducted later in the pregnancy. In amniocentesis, a doctor uses a hollow needle to enter the uterus—but unlike in CVS, the doctor removes a sample of amniotic fluid and not placental cells. Just as with CVS, the act of puncturing the uterus can cause the woman to miscarry in exceedingly rare cases: amniocentesis has a tenth to a third of a percent potential of causing a miscarriage.[26] Yet amniocentesis delays risk rather than averting it. Because the procedure is conducted between fifteen and twenty weeks of gestation, with delivery of results taking around two weeks, a woman may be prohibited from aborting her pregnancy should she receive problematic results.

Although CVS will provide results weeks earlier than amniocentesis, it once was thought that the predictive power of CVS results was not as accurate as those from amniocentesis. More recent research, however, indicates that both procedures' results equally prognosticate the likelihood of genetic defect in the fetus.[27] The trouble with CVS is that, in 1 to 2 percent of cases, the sample identifies "mosaicism"; the genetic material collected describes the placenta but not the fetus.[28] An amniocentesis must then be conducted to obtain information about the fetus only, exposing both the woman and fetus to a new test and its attendant risks.

Beyond their risks, how accurate are the results of CVS and amniocentesis? Test results should not provide false positives, incorrect indications that a fetus has a genetic condition when it really does not. Nor should the results mislead by reporting false negatives, wherein the test has missed finding that the fetus does have a genetic defect. CVS and amniocentesis correctly report that a fetus has Down Syndrome 99 percent of the time; for other genetic conditions, positive test results are more than 90 percent correct.[29] But genetic testing results provide false hope for 2 to 5 percent of pregnancies tested.[30] These are the missed cases, where the baby is born with a genetic condition for which the tests did not provide advance warning. And then there are a myriad of genetic or developmental problems for which no fetal or maternal test exists. Again, a hodgepodge of numbers. One in a hundred women would have a miscarriage from CVS. One in a hundred results might incorrectly say that the twins had a chromosomal abnormality, but two in a hundred results might falsely indicate that there was nothing wrong with the twins. Was the 1 percent risk of miscarriage worth the 2 percent risk of incorrect negative results? And would I abort twins if I received positive test results, which could be incorrect 1 percent of the time?

As I considered my options and crunched the numbers, I heard about a new type of "noninvasive" prenatal screening test (NIPT, pronounced "nip-tee"). These genetic tests were heavily marketed by their manufacturers to doctors and aggressively advertised to pregnant women. Unlike standard genetic testing methods for fetuses, a NIPT collects blood only from the woman and purports to detect and test fetal DNA circulating in the woman's blood.[31] The nifty NIPT does not require collecting fetal blood or amniotic fluid, so it poses no risk of miscarriage to the fetus. According to its own promotional materials, NIPT is highly accurate for indicating whether the fetus was at risk for chromosomal abnormality. Reviews of the NIPT, however, have called in doubt its promotions.[32] Promos are advertising, which has the purpose of convincing a consumer to purchase something. NIPTs were not (and still are not at the time of publication) regulated by the FDA, and the test's promotional materials also do not undergo governmental review for scientific precision.[33] Further, even if NIPTs are all they proport themselves to be, their ads are silent about the predictive power of these tests for multiple fetuses.

Taking a NIPT would provide me no needed information and only delay my receipt of reliable results that would indicate whether I should continue or terminate my pregnancy. NIPT screens the population of pregnant women for those with elevated risk of bearing a fetus with chromosomal abnormalities. Women indicated to be at higher risk are then supposed to be referred for further testing to confirm the screening results. I already knew of my elevated risk—this had been shown by the high nuchal translucency results seen on my ultrasound. Regardless of NIPT results, I would need to have an invasive prenatal genetic test to determine the likelihood that my fetuses had specific chromosomal abnormalities. If I wanted assurance of the genetic health of my fetuses, there was no way to avoid having a CVS or amniocentesis. My doctors and my good sense guided me away from taking a NIPT.

I chose to proceed with the CVS, accepting that there would be a slight chance that I would terminate the pregnancy based on erroneous testing results. An abortion would not be the end of my world or of my family; I could conceive again. I returned to the doctor who conducted the genetic tests for my first pregnancy. He had done more CVS than any other doctor on the East Coast, and my research showed that the best CVS outcomes were provided by a very experienced physician. The doctor's error rates were reportedly very low and his Yelp ratings very high.

In yet another darkened room, I drank a gallon of water to inflate my bladder to assist the ultrasound imaging, lay back on a paper-covered table, got covered in ultrasound goo, and waited for the needlestick. Then, I spent the rest of the day on my back with my feet in the air to ward off any uterine fluid leaks or muscle contractions that might lead to a miscarriage. Three days later, the rapid results came back, with a full genetic profile delivered within a week.

My fetuses' CVS results were the most encouraging news of my entire twin pregnancy: absolutely no problems were found. Accepting the slight chance that the tests missed something, I was comforted by the news. Genetically, at least, there was no cause to worry about the twins. The concerning nuchal translucency results were as my doctor had originally suspected: likely just another sign of TTTS.

Apparently, I was going to stay pregnant with two fetuses, at least for a while. It was likely that, because of TTTS, one or both would not survive. But for as long as they resided in me, I thought the twins should be named. I never intended these names to be permanent or used by others—perhaps like the twins themselves, the names would be known only to me. The CVS results gave us one other piece of important information: the sex of the fetuses. They were boys. Throwing out my long list of potential girls' names, which I had held over from my first pregnancy, I thought of the bigger fetus as Declan and the smaller one as Connor.

My goal was not to make the same mistake I had made with my first child and to name my twins something common. My first pregnancy was so routine and unremarkable that I gave birth with midwives in a nonhospitalized birthing center. The birthing center required all women due in the same month to meet every other week to discuss our prenatal care, birth plans, and breastfeeding goals. We never discussed the names we would give our babies, keeping these as highly guarded secrets. Nonetheless, and perhaps because we all were subtly influenced by the name of a TV character popular at the time,[34] five of the ten expectant mothers in my January cohort named their babies Finn.

I would do better this go-round, and I would be guided by statistics. The US Social Security Administration (SSA) publishes a website list of the top ten boys' and girls' names from the preceding year.[35] While this list will help parents avoid naming their child whatever was too popular last year, far more helpful is the SSA's change in popularity tool.[36] Using this tool helps to predict trends. Take my own name, Genevieve, as an example. Over the past eighteen years, Genevieve has leapt from the 502nd most popular girls' name to the 172nd most popular. Clearly, Genevieve is trending upward. Parents wishing to avoid a trendy name would do well to avoid it.

The SSA website showed the problem with naming the smaller twin Connor, should he survive. Connor has remained in the top fifty names for boys for the last two decades. A Connor would likely have other Connors in his class—and especially if he lived nearby. Consulting the SSA's Popular Names by State tool shows that Connor is popular not only in our district but also in the two neighboring states. We lived in a virtual hotbed of Connors! I grew even less enthusiastic when I cross-referenced the SSA results for Connor with those from a website that recorded the political party and educational attainment for all names recorded in the United States.[37] Apparently, most Connors are Republicans and only half have a college degree. Many had a gun in their homes. Naming my child Connor did not seem particularly auspicious. But given that my little Connor was unlikely ever to be listed on a birth certificate, there seemed no harm in giving him that name in utero.

Declan was more promising. Declan did not figure in the top thousand baby names for the past year, nationally or locally. Because it was so rare, the name was not shown to be trending up or down. The names and political party website found only four hundred Declans registered as voters in the entire United States. These Declans were mostly Democrats, two-thirds of them had a college degree, and relatively few were gun owners. Declan was a strong-sounding name for the bigger twin, even, again, if I had not planned to use it. Frankly, it was a little too unusual even for my taste.

Chapter Four

A Tail and a Burrito

My husband and I drove up to Johns Hopkins to meet the famous fetal surgeon who had responded to my email. We found his office space under construction and his secretary working out of a janitor's closet. He commandeered an entire operating theater to examine me, and a team of other fetal medicine specialists, medical residents, obstetricians, and sonographers filed in for the show. A screen was lowered across the room and a camera aimed at it. My uterus and its contents were magnified and displayed for all to see.

The doctor manipulated the ultrasound wands himself, instead of leaving the job to the sonographer. He narrated the projected images for the benefit of the other doctors assembled, who took notes throughout the lecture. Yes, there were two fetuses. One was much larger with a big pool of fluid around him. The smaller twin was tiny for his gestational age, and he was almost stuck to the wall of the uterus with an oblong fluid pocket surrounding him. The big fetus's sac of amniotic fluid was five times as large as his brother's sac. The membrane separating the twins' amniotic sacs appeared almost as a wispy, dashed line—almost as if the sacs were trying to merge.

Switching to a pulsed-wave, color-flow Doppler ultrasound machine, which uses the same technology as the meteorologists on the TV news use to track rainstorms, the doctor then traced the flow of blood from the placenta to each fetus. The other doctors in the room murmured and took notes as blue-and-red dots were superimposed over each fetus on display on the projector screen. With every heartbeat, the smaller, donor fetus pushed blood toward the placenta through the umbilical artery. The fetus's blood must reach the placenta to obtain fresh oxygen and nutrients from the mother. As TTTS worsens, the blood donor twin's heart becomes too weak to push its blood toward the placenta, and the blood becomes too thick to move. In severe TTTS cases, there may be no diastolic flow in the cord. Only an inadequate systolic flow occurs toward the placenta when the fetus's heart beats. The fetus is thus starved of oxygen and food and does not grow. If the systolic flow stops, the fetus succumbs.[1]

The little donor twin's tiny developing heart pressed on, with blood moving out to the placenta. It was not immediately obvious how blood was returning to the fetus, though. The blood vessel that should have returned oxygenated blood to the donor instead directed this blood to the recipient twin, who had his own problems. The recipient twin was being pumped full of his brother's blood, and his heart was straining to keep up. Already, there was evidence that the bigger twin's heart was forming incorrectly, with the heart valves struggling to process the flow of blood and the heart muscles weakening because the smaller twin was doing all the hard pumping work.

Fetal surgery for TTTS is based on two primary criteria: the relative size of the amniotic sacs around each twin and the blood flow in the twins' umbilical cords. Surgery is permitted before twenty weeks if the depth of fluid in the donor's amniotic sac depth is greater than or equal to eight centimeters and the fluid depth in the recipient's sac is less than or equal to two centimeters. In addition, before authorizing surgery, doctors will look for no blood flow or reversed blood flow from the mother's placenta to the donor fetus. The doctor informed me that I was not yet a candidate for surgery or other intervention for TTTS. My fetuses were only at eleven weeks of gestation, and the amniotic sac around the donor fetus was at 2.5 centimeters deep—but the fluid depth had not yet reached the critical level of only 2.1 centimeters.[2] Further, the donor's heart still was able to push blood forward toward the placenta. How blood was returning to the donor was somewhat of a mystery, but the doctor presumed that the fetuses' blood vessels had connected across their amniotic sacs, allowing the recipient to transfuse the donor with some of the oxygenated blood he received.

The doctor would have to monitor my situation closely, as TTTS can worsen rapidly. I would need to visit him at Hopkins once a week until I met the surgical criteria, which I would certainly reach soon. I would need to negotiate with my health insurance, to ensure it would pay for the surgery I would eventually require. I also would need to continue my visits with my obstetrician. The fetal specialist's job was to monitor the health of my fetuses but not to provide me with maternal healthcare. Carrying fetuses with TTTS was a risk to my own health, exposing me to stroke-inducing hypertension and pulmonary edema. Someone else would be responsible for trying to prevent me from suffering these outcomes.

My spouse and I began making the weekly, traffic-fighting, two-to-three-hour roundtrip trek to Hopkins. After handing off our toddler to a nanny, we'd eat breakfast in the car on the way up and have lunch on the road on the return. We tried to arrive at our offices in time to work at least six hours. But I still was working shortened days while I transitioned from my earlier maternity leave. My frequent absences from the office had been noted; my pregnancy situation needed a resolution—and soon.

There would be no forthcoming easy or quick fix. Each visit to the fetal specialist seemed to bring more bad news. The fluid levels in each fetus's amniotic sac remained highly discordant, above the 25 percent difference that was definitional for TTTS. The recipient twin's sac fluid depth was above eight centimeters, also matching TTTS criteria. The donor's fluid depth was too low, indicating that he was receiving scant nutrition and oxygen and urinating very little. But the donor's fluid levels remained two tenths of a centimeter above the level where the TTTS surgical protocols permitted intervention.

The donor twin had still other challenges beyond too little fluid in his amniotic sac. He was not growing, something the doctors attributed to selective intrauterine growth restriction (sIUGR). His umbilical cord only had two blood vessels instead of the usual three, limiting the amount of blood he could receive through it. And those two vessels were "marginally inserted" in the small placental share available to him. This meant that his cord functioned as if it had an electrical short in it, with a blood flow that flickered on and off, depending on his movement and that of his twin.

In a mono-di twin pregnancy sIUGR is—yet again for my pregnancy—an uncommon and fatal condition. It is relatively common (occurring in 15 percent of twin pregnancies) that even identical twin fetuses are different sizes. But a size difference of more than 15 percent between the fetuses is associated with an increased risk of death of both.[3] When one of the fetuses is very tiny, weighing less than the tenth percentile, and there is a resulting 25 percent weight difference between the twins, the pregnancy is considered to be complicated by sIUGR.[4] This condition is found in only 10 percent of monochorionic pregnancies of identical twins.[5] Whereas TTTS is caused by fetuses' oversharing of their blood supplies, sIUGR is caused by the fetuses' unequal sharing of the placenta. The smaller, growth-restricted twin has a smaller share of the placenta, which challenges the fetus's further growth and causes additional problems with its circulation. Blood flow through the smaller twin's umbilical artery toward the placenta is highly resistant and can stop or reverse.

Unlike TTTS, which causes adverse outcomes for both fetuses, sIUGR affects only the growth-restricted fetus. The larger fetus is not harmed by the twin's sIUGR per se, and a normally growing fetus is unaffected by his twin's inability to grow at a typical rate. sIUGR can have similar effects as TTTS, though, because the death of the smaller twin as a result sIUGR may cause neurodevelopmental problems for the larger twin. sIURG can be treated with cord coagulation of the smaller twin, killing that fetus. The choice to terminate the growth-restricted twin is intended to save the larger twin from death or brain damage in the event of the smaller twin's sudden fetal demise. As with TTTS, when to perform cord coagulation is the subject of medical debate, and the ideal timing for terminating the smaller fetus is unknown. Performing the cord coagulation in the wrong way or at the wrong time would subject the larger fetus to all the complications of an unmanaged death of the smaller twin.

TTTS and sIUGR were not the only problems my smaller twin faced. As noted earlier, the poor little fetus had only two blood vessels in an umbilical cord that should have had three. Normal umbilical cords have two arteries and one vein. In less than a half to one percent of pregnancies, though, the fetus's umbilical cord has one artery and one vein.[6] When two-vessel cords are found, usually the left artery is absent; oddly, my smaller fetus lacked his right umbilical artery. Two-vessel cords are not themselves problematic, but they are associated with sIUGR, unequal placental share, and genetic malformations.[7] The smaller fetus had fewer resources to assist his growth.

If the combination of TTTS, sIUGR, and a two-vessel cord weren't challenging enough, the smaller twin had one more strike against him: his compromised umbilical cord was marginally implanted into the tiny portion of the placenta he had been allotted. In "marginal implantation," the umbilical cord is implanted in the amnions but not fully into the placenta; its connection is supported by very little placental tissue.[8] Seventeen percent of twin pregnancies are complicated by marginal cord implantation for one of the fetuses.[9] Anomalous cord insertion doubles the risk the fetus will die before birth.[10] Should the fetus survive pregnancy, a marginal cord insertion is related to serious malformations, preterm birth, low birthweight, and lower Apgar scores for the baby.[11] For the mother, marginal cord implantation is correlated with preeclampsia and hypertension.[12]

The mixture of TTTS, sIUGR, and a two-vessel cord with marginal insertion was highly unusual and confounding for my doctors, who had never seen the confluence of these factors. The rare probability of such a combination challenges mathematics. The chances of an identical twin pregnancy are only three-tenths of a percent. Within those pregnancies with identical twins, TTTS is found 10 percent of the time, and sIUGR also occurs in 10 percent of mono-mono twin pregnancies. TTTS and sIUGR are often found together, but no one knows how often.[13] Up to 1 percent of pregnancies have fetuses with two-vessel cords, and an umbilical cord is marginally implanted in 17 percent of twin pregnancies. With apologies to the professors at my graduate school, my recollection of my education in biostatistics again fails me, but it seems to me that all these factors are found in only .005 percent of pregnancies.

The rare combination was also disastrous for my pregnancy. With only TTTS and with appropriate care, the fetuses might have a chance of survival. But TTTS complicated by sIUGR meant the possible interventions were fewer and the risks higher for both fetuses. Adding a two-vessel cord and marginal insertion to the mix of syndromes meant there was little possibility that the smaller twin would grow and develop. The little fetus would likely die, which would cause the larger twin to perish. For same-sex twins, if one dies between twenty and twenty-four gestational weeks, only 8 percent of cotwins survive. The Hopkins team joked that each time I visited, I received worse information than the week before, but that I took it all so well and so cheerfully. What choice did I have? Crying wouldn't have solved the many medical mysteries I faced. Instead, I poured myself into researching each condition and its potential treatments.

I had earned a reputation around Hopkins for being slightly difficult and demanding, challenging whatever presumptions the medical team made and bringing printouts of medical journal articles to my appointments. I corrected the sonographer when she incorrectly used the term "gender" rather than "sex" when she wondered whether I knew if my fetuses were boys or girls. "Gender is a social construct," I snippily informed the ultrasound tech. Whether the twins were masculine or feminine would not be known for many years, but I had received the results of their chromosomal test, which said that the twins were male.

When my doctor told me that, in addition to all his other problems, the smaller twin appeared to have a tail, it was par for the course. It might be a sign of a neural tube defect such as spina bifida, but no one could be certain until and if the child was born. Nothing could be done about this information, and no treatment offered to the fetus. Had there been only one fetus to contend with, perhaps we could have been explored doing fetal surgery to correct a potential neural tube defect. But with his bloodstream connected to an identical twin, most interventions were out of the question for the smaller twin. Any disruption of the little twin would terminate the larger twin. All I could do was accept the information, investigate its outcomes, suggest any alternative scenarios the research indicated, and move on.

Spina bifida is, like everything else that was occurring with my pregnancy, rare but not uncommon. Occurring in up to two thousand in every four million pregnancies, spina bifida happens when the brain, spinal cord, or their protective covering does not fully develop.[14] Depending on the severity of the malformation and whether the spinal cord is exposed through an opening in the spine, a child with spina bifida may have few symptoms or complete paralysis with urinary and fecal incontinence. A tail visualized on a fetal ultrasound may be an early warning sign of an improperly formed vertebrae in the spine, pointing to potential problems with the lower spinal cord and motor control of the legs, bladder, and bowel.

There was still more. "I see a spot in the little twin's stomach," the doctor informed me at a visit that had otherwise gone well. "He could have eaten a burrito, or it could be his parasitic triplet."

For once, the timing was impeccable. The *Washington Post* had just weeks before published an article about fetus in fetu, or parasitic twins and triplets.[15] The news reported on a then current and several historical cases of children being born with stable abdominal lumps that mostly remained the same size. These lumps differ from teratomas, which are also common in infants and are growing tumors containing different cell types, including, famously, hair and teeth.[16] When excised, the fetus in fetu masses were found to hold arms, legs, and even heads. They were from the semideveloped twins or triplets that had been absorbed by the baby's body while in utero. Provided that the parasitic twin's remains were removed from the infant, she or he would suffer no ill effect and would have a normal childhood.[17]

When a twin or triplet does not survive pregnancy, the usual outcome—more common than fetus in fetu—is that the mother's body absorbs the fetus. The miscarriage and reabsorption of a twin or triplet fetus is called vanishing twin syndrome.[18] For pregnancies as advanced as mine, beyond the first trimester, miscarrying a twin or triplet could result in the mother's hemorrhaging, infection, and preterm labor.[19] If the smaller twin (with his parasitic triplet) were to die, the results could be dangerous for both the larger twin and for me.

Two visits to Hopkins later, the spot—whatever it was—had disappeared from the smaller twin. We concluded that the doctor had been correct with his initial presumption. The little twin likely had merely made a Taco Bell run and eaten a burrito. Whatever the mass was in his stomach was no cause for concern.

Concern remained about the smaller twin's risk for spina bifida, but fortunately, human beings are unlikely to be born with tails. A lower back protrusion seen on ultrasound usually reabsorbs into the body, although if the tail is a sign of spina bifida, neurological problems may remain. A review of medical literature over the past few decades found few recorded instances of children with tails.[20] Yet with my luck with this pregnancy, my child would make history as the first example of a human with a prehensile tail.

(*Chapter Five*)

Announcements and Complaints

My supervisor was getting suspicious about the amount of time I was taking each week for medical appointments. Every Monday, my husband and I would schlep to Baltimore, where I would submit to another ultrasound complete with Doppler. We would then speed back to our jobs in DC. We didn't expect the pregnancy to result in a baby or babies, so we had mentioned it to no one.

However, I was looking more and more bloated. Thanks to an exceptionally cold winter with an incursion of the polar vortex from the far north, I had hidden my expanded size under layers of bulky clothes. My entire extended family, who had bunked with me in a hotel room for a weekend in February, hadn't noticed a thing. My condition would soon become obvious, however, even to the oblivious. My spouse and I thought it wise to say something to our families and close friends.

When I was sixteen weeks pregnant, we drafted an email announcing the pregnancy and its likely impending loss. We sent the email to twenty people, including our parents.

Dear family and friends,
We wanted to let you know that GG is pregnant with twins, who are due in August. Unfortunately, the twins are very sick with the condition called twin-to-twin transfusion syndrome.[1] It is unlikely that both will survive, and it is possible neither will. We are seeking medical care to try to improve the odds.
We had been delaying announcing the pregnancy in the hopes of having more certain (and happy) news to share.

Please forgive us if we do not send out lots of updates or wish to discuss the situation. But we appreciate your keeping us in your thoughts and, ultimately, will let you know how things turn out.

Surprisingly, our families were amazingly understanding. Although both sets of parents called my spouse to ask for more details, blessedly, none called me. I was dreading a conversation with my parents, which I feared was inevitable. During my first pregnancy, my mother had made eminently clear her views on pregnancy termination for any reason. She had said that she would prefer that I die in childbirth than that I seek an abortion.

My mom's no abortion, no exceptions opinion is one shared by many people—but not the majority—in the United States. In 2021, 39 percent of Americans (and 43 percent of Catholics, my mother's demographic) said that abortion should be prohibited in all or most cases.[2] In contrast, 59 percent (and 55 percent of Catholics) said that abortion should be legal in all or most cases.[3] Following enactment of state laws that would ban all abortions for any reason within four weeks of a woman's last menstrual period, American support for abortion rose to its highest level in two decades. In July 2019, those who opposed abortion in all or most cases dropped to a record low, 36 percent.[4] Although men and women support and oppose abortion in equal numbers,[5] the increased backing for access to abortion care is from growth in support from female voters who identify as independents or Democrats, often described as progressive or liberal.[6] Among Republicans, who tend to be more conservative voters, 52 percent believe that abortion should always or usually be illegal.[7]

American support for abortion depends on the circumstance. A poll in 2018 presented several hypothetical pregnancy scenarios and inquired about support for each. During the first three months of pregnancy, 83 percent of respondents would support availability of abortion when the expectant mother's life was in danger.[8] Sixty-seven percent would permit aborting the pregnancy when the child would be born with a life-threatening illness, and 56 percent would support a woman's choice to abort if the child were to be born mentally disabled.[9]

When a pregnancy was more advanced, public support for abortion was still robust, at 75 percent, when the woman's life was in danger.[10] But only 35 percent would support abortion in the final trimester of pregnancy if the child were to be born mentally disabled.[11] Forty-eight percent would permit aborting the pregnancy if the child were to be born with a life-threatening illness.[12]

Now, my stakes in needing all pregnancy options, including abortion, were higher than they had been during my first pregnancy. I had a toddler who was utterly reliant on me, to the point that his life was sustained, in part, by my breast milk. My pregnancy was threatening my health, at least one of my children would likely be born with life-threatening illnesses, and it was probable that the other child would be mentally disabled. Termination was a reasonable resolution to the problem. Instead of spending all my time, money, and emotional well-being fighting to save two very sick fetuses, I could devise a polite story of pregnancy loss and abort. I still was on the fence as to how to proceed, but my family left me in peace to process my decision.

Announcement of the pregnancy went less smoothly at my work. My employer-provided health insurance is gold-plated and covers virtually every medical procedure imaginable. Acupuncture, chiropractors, massage, Lasik, and all manner of therapies are approved services. But what about abortion? Or fetal surgery? I checked with my health insurance administrator to inquire.

Over several calls and emails, and despite my insistence, my health plan administrator would not tell me what coverage I had for pregnancy interventions. Each time I asked, she seemed flustered by my questions. Instead of answering me, and knowing nothing of my own religious convictions, she suggested that I "trust in Jesus." She also said she would pray for me. Unhelpful. I'd have to figure out this conundrum on my own, yet again. Unraveling which services my health insurance covered required determining what sort of insurance plan I had, how that plan was affected—if at all—by US federal and local law, what was considered the standard of care for TTTS treatment, and whether the health insurance plan recognized that standard of care in its benefits determination. Thank goodness I was a lawyer.

My employer self-insures the healthcare of its employees through a plan that is administered by Aetna, a large private insurance company. Because it is offered in the United States, my employer's health insurance plan still must comply with the standards set out in the Affordable Care Act, also known as Obamacare. Before implementation of a provision of Obamacare in 2014, maternity care was not a required benefit of US insurance plans. Only 12 percent of private insurance plans sold to individuals included coverage of medical costs for pregnancy, labor, delivery, and newborn baby care.[13] Maternity coverage had to be added as a costly rider to the plans that did not cover it. But because insurers could consider pregnancy as a preexisting condition, women who were already pregnant were barred from purchasing maternity care riders or enrolling in insurance plans that covered pregnancy and delivery costs.

Thankfully, by the time I was pregnant with my twins in 2015, Obamacare had taken effect and mandated that maternity coverage was one of ten essential health benefits to be covered by all health insurance plans offered to individuals, families, and small groups. My insurance included coverage for prenatal screening tests, which paid for the costs of my weekly ultrasounds at Hopkins. Although my insurance required a 20 percent copay for all medical procedures, my plan also included a cap on out-of-pocket costs, including my copay. I found out that I was pregnant in January; by February, my ultrasound costs had exceeded the out-of-pocket cost cap. The insurance picked up the full cost of my scans thereafter.

Though medically necessary maternity care must be covered, the Obamacare law gives private insurers discretion in determining the types of procedures they will pay for and what is considered "medically necessary." For most insurers, "medically necessary" includes those medical procedures that are the standard of care for the condition in question. These best standard practices are distinguished from procedures that insurers consider "experimental," which are not covered under the insurance plan.

Professional medical groups issue practice bulletins that help doctors and insurers define what is the best standard of care versus what is still experimental. The Society of Maternal-Fetal Medicine (SMFM) has clinical guidance that instructs that laser fetal surgery should be offered to patients with pregnancies complicated by severe TTTS.[14] Recognizing that laser fetal surgery is available only at a few locations worldwide, the society further instructs that less effective therapies (expectant management and amnioreduction) be provided to patients who cannot travel to receive laser surgery.[15] Aetna, my insurance administrator, agrees with the society about what is medically necessary for the treatment of TTTS. Aetna's clinical policy guidelines for its insurance coverage say, "Aetna considers in utero fetal surgery medically necessary for any of the following indications [including] . . . laser ablation or occlusion of anastomotic vessels in early, severe twin-twin transfusion syndrome."[16] Should it become necessary, and if my pregnancy qualified for it, my health insurance would have covered laser surgery for TTTS in 2015.

Determining my insurance coverage for abortion was more complicated. Federal Obamacare standards for health insurance leave to each state determinations of whether to permit insurers to cover abortion care, and the federal public health insurance for the poor, Medicaid, does not cover abortion at all. In many states, even if the employer wanted to and the insurer would otherwise allow it, health insurance plans may not cover the costs of a pregnancy termination. Eleven states prohibit insurance coverage for abortion in all private insurance plans written in the state, including those plans that are offered under Obamacare.[17] Twenty-two states prohibit abortion coverage in certain health insurance plans, such as those that are given to public employees, including public school teachers, firefighters, police officers, and state government bureaucrats.[18] In the states that prevent insurers from paying for abortion costs, two states maintain this prohibition for public employees even when the pregnancy endangers the mother's life.[19] In Idaho, Indiana, Kansas, Kentucky, Michigan, Missouri, Nebraska, North Dakota, and Oklahoma, if a woman is dying in pregnancy and requires an abortion to save her life, the woman must purchase at additional cost a separate insurance plan rider so that her health insurer can defray some of the abortion's costs.[20]

Fortunately, I did not live in one of those nine states. My insurer could cover a pregnancy termination if the insurance plan I signed up for included abortion as a covered benefit. According to the Society of Maternal-Fetal Medicine, an abortion might be medically necessary, especially in a complicated case like mine. In its TTTS clinical guidance, the society said: "In cases complicated by severe unequal placental sharing with marked discordant growth and IUGR [inter-uterine growth restriction], major malformation affecting one twin, or evidence of brain injury either before or subsequent to laser, selective reduction by cord occlusion or by termination of the entire pregnancy may be reasonable management choices for the patient and her family."[21] My insurance policy's very small print left that reasonable management choice to me. Tucked away under covered benefits in a paragraph of services related to maternity care, prenatal tests, contraception, and infertility treatment was "pregnancy termination." No restrictions were listed, no footnotes appended.

I could end my pregnancy at any time I saw fit, and my insurance would cover that cost.

More recently, a wrinkle has been added to the determination of whether an employer-provided health insurance plan would cover fetal laser surgery to treat TTTS. If a woman's employer opposes health interventions on moral or religious grounds, the employer could block its employees' health insurance plan from paying for these services. In 2017, the Trump administration issued a new health insurance regulation that allows any employer, nonprofit or for-profit, to claim a religious objection to providing insurance coverage for certain healthcare and to exclude that care from the health insurance plans it sponsors.[22] A different regulation allows any employer that is not a publicly traded company to refuse to provide health insurance coverage to services to which the employer morally objects.[23] The original purpose of these regulations was to allow employers to prohibit their employees' access to contraception through workplace health insurance plans.[24] Employers have interpreted these regulations broadly to withhold insurance coverage of infertility treatment, gender reassignment surgery, and hormonal therapies. In late 2019 federal courts temporarily blocked the enforcement of the new regulations, buying more time for those who relied on their employer-provided health insurance.[25] Finally, in the summer of 2020, the US Supreme Court upheld the Trump administration's regulations, cutting off millions of Americans from a wide array of reproductive and other health services.[26]

Had these regulations been in place in 2015, they could have been used to block me from receiving either fetal surgery or abortion care. When I asked my health insurer administrator about covered services under my insurance plan, she refused to identify these services and instead suggested I rely on divine intervention to resolve my medical needs. The administrator clearly had religious and moral beliefs that affected her willingness to assist me. I had to use my own skills and education to determine the extent of my insurance coverage. My health insurance plan administrator could not stop me from receiving the services listed in my plan or my insurer from paying for those services.

Now, my administrator may be on stronger legal ground to seek to deny me insurance coverage for fetal surgery or abortion. We work at an organization that is not a publicly traded company, so the administrator could claim either a religious or moral objection to providing me information about certain of my health insurance plan benefits. She would have no obligation to refer me to others in the organization who could answer my questions; she could simply block my access to my plan information. Because she is the liaison between the employees and our health insurance company, she also could insist that the insurer not pay for or reimburse me for bills related to fetal surgery or abortion. It would be possible that I would learn that my claims were not reimbursable after I incurred thousands of dollars of costs. My employer's representative could wield ultimate financial power over my receipt of healthcare that was lifesaving, appropriate, and gold standard—but that she found objectionable.

Someone—or someones—at my work complained to my boss about my pregnancy. The complainants were never identified to me, but the substance of their concerns was communicated, as was the fact that I was being investigated. First, I was accused of not being collegial and friendly about my pregnancy. Specifically, my accuser said that I had refused to discuss my pregnancy when asked about it. Additionally, I was alleged to have pushed away a co-worker's hand when, in the elevator and uninvited by me, she tried to pat my protruding belly. To these accusations, I pled guilty. I was deeply ambivalent about my pregnancy because I expected its outcome to be sad and potentially debilitating. I hid the pregnancy for as long as possible at work and ignored pointed comments about my recent weight gain. When my condition became noticeable, my colleagues wanted to chitchat about it. I shut down these conversations as quickly as possible, saying that the fetus was sick and that I didn't want to discuss it further. Because I worked on the ninth floor, my approach made for some long and awkward elevator rides.

My organization has few Americans in it and operates by different cultural norms than the standard US workplace. Personal space during interactions is much less than most Americans would find comfortable, with people standing much closer than is customary for us. Common conversational topics too are beyond the realm of what is considered polite to an American, with workplace colleagues finding it appropriate to comment on each other's appearance, weight, size, shape, and plans for marriage and childbearing. Combining these two cultural eccentricities is the practice of patting an expectant woman's belly; at my organization, an entire elevator of people might pat and rub a pregnant woman as they exit. In other cultures, this is a perfectly normal expression of a wish of good luck to the woman. To an American—or to me—it feels like an assault.

The second complaint about me was that my pregnancy made others feel uncomfortable. Perhaps I wasn't as joyous as I should be about being pregnant. Or maybe there were no other women at my job level who were pregnant. My coworkers in management were all men or older women who had not had children; generally, only the secretaries and junior staff were ever observed to be pregnant. Whatever the reason, my colleagues were discomfited by my lumbering, waddling, distended pregnant body and my unsmiling face and relayed their distress to my supervisor.

Workplace pregnancy discrimination was once so commonplace that it was accepted and unremarkable. Responding to female US presidential candidate Elizabeth Warren's reminiscences of being fired because she was pregnant, thousands of women have told similar stories on social media.[27] When she was pregnant with me in the late 1970s, my own mother was fired from her job as a TV news editor in Detroit, Michigan. The predominant view was that it was embarrassing to have a visibly pregnant woman in the workplace, and employers presumed that the woman would not return to work after having her baby, anyway. My mom's sacking was perfectly compliant with the laws at that time: the Supreme Court had found in 1976 that employers' discrimination against pregnant women did not violate civil rights protections.[28]

In 1978, the US Congress passed the Pregnancy Discrimination Act (PDA), which prohibits employers with more than fifteen employees from discriminating against a worker on the basis of pregnancy, childbirth, or related medical conditions.[29] An employer cannot refuse to hire a woman because she is pregnant or because of the prejudices of coworkers against pregnant women. The law also forbids employers from treating a pregnant worker differently from any other worker when it comes to any other aspect of employment, including pay, job assignments, promotions, training, and firing. US courts have interpreted the PDA as requiring employers to provide pregnant workers reasonable accommodations to do their jobs.[30]

The PDA is routinely violated by the employers to which it applies and routinely ignored by the employers that do not need to comply with it. Each year, the Equal Employment Opportunity Commission (EEOC) resolves in the workers' favor thousands of complaints of pregnancy discrimination.[31] Employers illegally continue to take job opportunities away from pregnant workers or to fire women on maternity leave or to pass over for promotions those who have recently given birth. In workplaces like mine that are not covered by the PDA or any US labor law, employees have no legal recourse when their employer institutes an adverse human resources action against them for looking pregnant at work—or for not being sufficiently smiley and chatty about gestating a difficult pregnancy.

I received a talking-to from my boss about my poor attitude and the need to improve it, and I was instructed to smooth over my office relationships with my colleagues. I also was referred for management counseling. My department contracted with a business coach from the private sector for this purpose. Blessedly, the coach was a woman who never had children but was an American with long experience in large US businesses. She interviewed me and conducted a thorough review of the complaints against me, interviewing my accusers as well. She then delivered her findings to me and to my boss: I had done nothing wrong, and my organization's censuring me because of the complaints it received would have been barred by US law had that law applied to my organization. My employer had its own policies and rules about gender equality and prohibitions about firing workers on maternity leave, but these had never been interpreted as providing employees protections against discrimination or coworker bias based on pregnancy. Essentially, my workplace was like the pre-PDA United States.

The coach also met with me privately. She inquired: How many weeks of maternity leave would I have with my organization? How many weeks of vacation had I banked? What other leave would apply to me? She advised me, "Have your babies. Take your maternity leave, your vacation, your sick leave, every last minute. And then get another job. There is nothing here for you."

Chapter Six

Scopes and Interventions

The amniotic fluid depths around my twins remained just outside the levels necessary for a formal TTTS diagnosis, which would have opened the door to me for treatment. The pocket of fluid around the big twin was around ten centimeters, an amount that exceeded even the conservative criterion for TTTS. More recent medical guidance provides a cutoff of six centimeters for the deepest pocket before eighteen weeks of gestation,[1] a level I far surpassed. But the fluid depth around the smaller twin was 2.3 centimeters. For TTTS, the fluid around the donor twin had to be less than 2.1 centimeters. Yet the smaller twin was not growing and was at only 3 percent of his expected weight for gestational age. Fitting within the TTTS picture, the larger twin was many times larger than the smaller, although growth discordance between the fetuses is not itself a diagnostic criterion for TTTS.[2] The donor twin also continued to pump away his blood to his brother, but a return blood flow was seen only intermittently, if at all.

Although I did not meet the strict clinical definition of TTTS, my doctor made an executive decision to label my pregnancy as complicated by TTTS. With this diagnosis, I had three potential resolutions for my pregnancy. I was now at sixteen weeks, and I needed to act quickly, as the time was growing short to avail myself of any of the choices. As a first option, I could abort both fetuses. Or the doctor could use a laser to cauterize the umbilical cord of the smaller, donor fetus. As a third option, the doctor could try to save both fetuses.

I was midway through my second trimester, but the fetuses were not yet viable. An abortion of fetuses of this size was beyond the capability of most freestanding abortion clinics, such as those run by Planned Parenthood. But one still could be procured at various hospitals and a specialty abortion clinic for second and third trimester terminations.

As an alternative to aborting both fetuses, cord coagulation, or cauterizing the umbilical cord of the donor fetus, offered a tantalizing possibility of producing one neurologically normal child. For this option, I still would need to have a difficult uterine surgery. The doctor would attempt to pierce the amniotic sac of the recipient twin in two locations to allow a scope access to the donor twin's umbilical cord. Then, through the scope, the doctor would use a laser to close off the umbilical cord of the donor, leading to his eventual death. If I delivered the surviving twin, I would also deliver the remains of the deceased fetus.

The cord coagulation option was not ideal for several reasons. The donor twin's umbilical cord was located toward the back of my uterus, making it tricky to access. The only route to it was through the recipient twin's amniotic sac. The laser would need to enter and exit the larger twin's sac, creating two holes and two opportunities for rupturing the membrane. With a ruptured amniotic sac, I would miscarry both twins. My anterior placenta could separate, putting me at greater risk of hemorrhage from the surgery. A hemorrhage would also cause a miscarriage. Further, because the recipient twin already showed signs of heart damage, it was conceivable that he had already suffered brain damage. Coagulating his twin's cord might serve to terminate the donor but not to produce a healthy recipient.

As a third option, the doctor could try to save both fetuses. The standard treatment for TTTS is to perform intrauterine surgery between the pregnancy's sixteenth and twenty-sixth week. A fetal surgeon fishes a hollow tube into the woman's uterus and then threads tiny cameras and lasers to cauterize the blood vessels that lead from one twin's amniotic sac to the other. Each of these tools—the scopes (which also can have surrounding sheaths), the cameras, and the lasers—must be approved for the surgeries where their use is intended. Without the permission of both a regulatory and an ethical body, the surgeon, no matter her skill or her desire, may not use tools in a surgical procedure.

In the United States, the Food and Drug Administration approves medical devices that are inserted into the body. The FDA has three levels of review before a device may ever be brought to market.[3] At the lowest level, the device manufacturer merely registers and lists the device with the FDA. Next is a premarket notification, in which the device manufacturer must show that the device is substantially equivalent in its manufacturing and performance

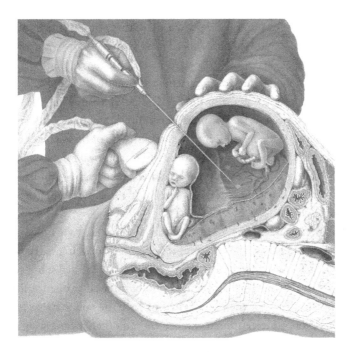

Fetal surgery of TTTS Twins. From Marjolijn S. Spruijt, Enrico
Lopriore, Sylke J. Steggerda, Femke Slaghekke, and Jeanine M. M.
Van Klink, "Twin-Twin Transfusion Syndrome in the Era of Feto-
scopic Laser Surgery: Antenatal Management, Neonatal Outcome and
Beyond," *Expert Review of Hematology* 13, no. 3 (2020): 259–67, 261,
fig. 7, https://www.tandfonline.com/doi/full/10.1080/17474086.2020
.1720643. Reprinted by permission of the publisher Taylor & Francis,
Ltd. (www.tandfonline.com).

to another device that has long been on the market or that the FDA has already reviewed. A higher level of scrutiny, called premarket approval (PMA),
is given to new devices that pose a significant risk of illness or injury. The
FDA requires clinical data to show a high-risk device's safety and efficacy. To
collect the data necessary to obtain a PMA, device manufacturers can apply
to the FDA for an exemption to permit the device's use in a clinical study. All
investigational studies must be first approved by an institutional review board
(IRB); in most cases, FDA approval also is required.

When I was pregnant, there were two alternative two-millimeter-diameter fetoscopes available for surgeries to address twin-to-twin transfusion syndrome. (A different scope could be used if we chose to coagulate the umbilical cord of the smaller twin in an attempt to save his brother.) One was for a posterior placenta, attached in the back of the uterus toward the woman's spine, and the other was for an anterior placenta, attached at the front of the uterus. Because I had an anterior placenta, only one of these scopes could be used on me. Both the scopes had a special FDA approval for exceptional use in TTTS surgery only. FDA approval had not been sought—nor had it been given—for using the scopes for laser surgery for selective intrauterine growth restriction alone.

Although he believed he should operate to separate the twins' blood vessels, my doctor insisted that "the law" prohibited him from doing so. In his view, full-blown TTTS—meeting all the diagnostic criteria, including for fluid depths—needed to develop before he would be allowed to operate using the only scopes available for the procedure. But once the donor twin's amniotic fluid levels dropped .2 centimeters more and all other criteria were met for him to make a TTTS diagnosis, my doctor could use the scopes to perform fetal surgery. With formally diagnosed TTTS present, the scopes then could be used to resolve other coexisting conditions, including sIUGR, that complicated the pregnancy.

In fact, the law did not prohibit my doctor from operating. The FDA does not restrict medical procedures because it does not regulate the practice of medicine. Once the FDA approves a device, the circumstances under which the device may be used are written on the device's label. Just because a label does not list a possible use of the device does not mean that use is proscribed. A doctor may use a device for reasons other than those for which the device was approved. If the doctor, based on her experience and knowledge, believes using a device in an "off label" manner could have positive outcomes for the patient, then that doctor may legally proceed, even if the use is not specified on the device's label. However, for devices that have an FDA-approved use but that would be used for something other than for what they were approved, a hospital's IRB must first approve that use if it would be considered experimental and involves human subjects.[4] In an emergency, the IRB ruling could be post hoc, after the surgery was completed.

When TTTS is combined with sIUGR, unequal placental share, and a two-vessel umbilical cord with marginal insertion, the combination of pregnancy complications is so rare that the scopes used perform surgery must be used off-label and for a reason other than only to address TTTS. Nevertheless, according to my doctor, Hopkins's IRB was unlikely to approve my case for fetal surgery. From the viewpoint of the hospitals, lawsuits can be avoided by only permitting the use of a device that is consistent with its label. Although I had chosen the risks associated with fetal surgery, including the risk that one or both of my fetuses would die during the operation, my doctor explained that the hospital feared that I would change my mind with an adverse surgical outcome and sue. That both my spouse and I were lawyers, one of us specializing in litigation and the other in healthcare, did not add to Hopkins's level of comfort. To convince Hopkins to let my doctor proceed, the scopes' labels would need to be revised or an exception to their labeled use found.

The device's manufacturer is responsible for proposing a label amendment to the FDA and for getting that revised label approved. Reams of data must support a request to revise a label, and the manufacturer has little incentive to conduct the studies to collect this data. In many instances, and especially when charges for different tools used in medical procedures are bundled together, health insurers will pay for off-label use of drugs or devices. From the manufacturer's perspective, there is no financial justification to spend the effort or money trying to change a label. The FDA process for a label change can take months—wasted time with little return on the investment.

I could only try to induce the manufacturer to provide the Hopkins IRB with the information it would require to permit my surgery. I had friends at the FDA who explained the agency's regulatory process to me and who found documentation for the manufacturer of the scopes used for fetal laser ablations. I called and wrote Storz, the manufacturer, to plead my case for relabeling.

There was hope! The FDA had designated Storz fetoscopes as humanitarian use devices (HUDs), and Storz had received approval from the FDA for a humanitarian device exemption (HDE) for its fetoscopes.[5] A humanitarian use device is intended to benefit patients whose condition is so rare that it manifests in no more than eight thousand individuals in the United States per year. Borderline TTTS combined with sIUGR and several other conditions clearly qualified, affecting only tens of American women per year. Having an HDE meant that Storz was exempt from having to collect as much data about the effectiveness of its devices and that the FDA had approved Storz scopes for use in rare fetal surgeries. Even with the HDE, all roads led back to the hospital IRB. After HDE approval, a HUD can be used only after an IRB also has approved its use.[6] Hospital IRBs may give blanket approval for certain HUD devices or may require case-by-case approval. Because TTTS surgery risks terminating the entire pregnancy, my doctor said, Hopkins's IRB's sanction was required for any fetal surgery operation that would use the Storz scopes.

IRBs review proposed medical experiments and research on people to ensure these are ethical. What is ethical is determined by an IRB's interpretation of a voluntary code adhered to by every doctor and of certain laws and regulations that control research funded by the US government. The American Medical Association's ethical code states that patients have the right to be treated with "courtesy, respect, dignity, and timely, responsive attention to his or her needs."[7] The patient's privacy and confidentiality must be maintained by all medical personnel. The doctor must provide the patient information about the benefits, risks, and costs of treatment alternatives and of forgoing treatment. Although the physician will offer guidance on the optimal course of action, the patient will decide whether to receive the care the physician recommends.

Medical ethics differ somewhat from research ethics. The FDA defines research ethics as demanding that experimental procedures protect the rights and welfare and ensure the informed consent of the "human subjects" of that research.[8] A human subject is not only the patient the doctor or surgeon proposes to treat with procedure, protocol, or medication; the subject is any "healthy human" or patient who is or becomes a participant in research, either as a recipient of a test procedure or medication or as a control.[9] Significantly for any pregnant patient, IRBs will consider the effect of the experiment on the fetus, regardless of the woman's informed consent to the procedure. In contravention of an ACOG Ethics Committee Opinion, the FDA now requires that the fetus's father must also give his consent for the pregnant mother to receive an experimental treatment that would benefit the fetus.[10]

The Trump administration FDA issued new guidance to IRBs on ethical considerations for clinical trials and human subjects research on pregnant women.[11] This guidance applies to FDA-regulated research the rules for clinical trials supported or conducted by the US Department of Health and Human Services. To be approved, a research therapy provided to a pregnant person must hold the possibility of direct benefit for the woman or the developing fetus. If there is no such benefit and if the research poses a risk to the fetus, that risk must be minimal and the least possible for achieving the objectives of an experiment that cannot be accomplished any other way. A minimal risk is one that is not greater than that ordinarily encountered in daily life or during a routine examination or test. (It is unclear whether ordinary risks are those from the normal, daily life of the woman or of her fetus, who is not yet alive.) When an IRB considers whether to approve research involving pregnant women, it should consider only those risks and benefits resulting from doing the research as opposed to doing nothing.

The FDA's elevation of a nonviable fetus to a having all the rights of a human research subject—and rights that exceed those even of the pregnant patient—may be intended charitably to protect the doctor and hospital from lawsuits. After all, the Institute of Medicine warned in 1994 that a woman's informed consent to participate in a clinical study may not be adequate to protect a study sponsor from liability for an injured fetus.[12] But prioritizing potential life over a fully grown woman—with her own aspirations and responsibilities—is a political decision to remove from consideration a woman's needs as well as wants. Abortion is painted as a wrong, not as a choice; thus, I was wrong for even being open to ending one fetus's life to preserve the other. Indeed, a whiff of abortion stigma and political maneuvering pervades the FDA's guidance on research involving pregnant women. The guidance states that individuals engaged in research on pregnant women will have no part in any decisions as to the timing, method, or procedures used to terminate a pregnancy.[13] No inducements can be offered to the pregnant woman to terminate her pregnancy. The agency warns that researchers engaged in the study or investigation with the pregnant subject "will have no part in determining the viability of a neonate."[14]

Guidance like this put me in a disadvantaged position with the IRB. My doctor and I were requesting permission for an experimental procedure that would benefit one fetus but would likely pose a risk to the other fetus. The doctor who would be conducting the laser surgery was the only one at

Hopkins who had the ability to do this surgery, but the timing, methods, and procedures he would use might result in the termination of one of the fetuses—and in the salvation of the other. If we did not intervene in the pregnancy, we would avoid the significant but uncertain risks attendant to surgery, but we would assume the significant but uncertain risks of doing nothing for a pregnancy complicated by multiple potentially fatal conditions.

There were no studies we could point to that offered guidance for my situation. At that time, the American Society for Maternal-Fetal Medicine still regarded laser surgery intervention in TTTS with suspicion, finding that meta-analysis data show no significant survival or neurological outcomes because of it.[15] In 2016, a year too late for me, a team of scientists conducted a meta-analysis of all available and reliable trials of interventions in "early" TTTS on which the criteria for intervention (that is, the depth of the amniotic fluid pockets and blood flows to the babies) were barely met.[16] The search for TTTS Stage I pregnancies to review found only 511 pregnancies, of which twin survival was studied in a mere 433 pregnancies.[17] Twin survival in fifty-one TTTS pregnancies treated with laser surgery was compared to seventy-three TTTS pregnancies in which no intervention was made. The researchers also examined using laser surgery proactively, as a first line treatment when TTTS was first suspected.

The early TTTS meta-analysis was a day late and a dollar short when I needed it, in 2015. Because of the rarity of TTTS, especially TTTS complicated by a myriad of factors, and the very few good reliable studies of the condition, my medical team had to draw their conclusions from an utter paucity of evidence. All we had to guide us were the outcomes of eleven TTTS Stage I pregnancies in which doctors had focused on the short-term survival and neurological health of the babies born.[18] And we had a retrospective review (not a gold-standard clinical study) that found that, for Stage I TTTS, laser surgery made no difference in the gestational age at delivery or the twins' survival immediately after delivery.[19] But we had nothing regarding the interaction of TTTS with sIUGR or the long-term neurological outcomes for sIUGR twins who had been separated by fetal laser coagulation. Realizing it was akin to a Hail Mary of a shot at the buzzer, my doctor submitted my case, his recommendations, and the Storz HDE to the Johns Hopkins IRB.

Lawyers know they have conclusively won or lost a case when a jury returns quickly with its verdict. By that standard, Johns Hopkins overwhelmingly rejected my argument for laser surgery. Within three days and relying on a cramped view of "ethics" that limited my care, the IRB denied my doctor's request to perform surgery to cauterize the blood vessels that led from the donor twin to the recipient twin. I did not meet the clinical criteria for TTTS, and laser ablation for sIUGR was deemed too experimental with too much risk for pregnancy loss and too little proven benefit. Hopkins was unwilling to let my surgeon try to save both fetuses with laser surgery, and I was unwilling to sacrifice one through cord coagulation. There was nothing more my doctor could do. He discharged me back to my high-risk obstetrician, wished me well, and told me to call if my situation changed.

(*Chapter Seven*)

Edge of Science

I f Hopkins couldn't help me, perhaps another hospital's IRB would make a different decision in my case. The question was where. From my initial research on TTTS, I knew of several doctors affiliated with US hospitals that had begun to offer laser surgery when a TTTS diagnosis was confirmed. Respected institutions, such as Children's Hospital of Philadelphia, Children's Hospital Los Angeles, University of Texas Medical School at Houston, and Children's Hospital Colorado, had affiliated with physicians who had authored the TTTS studies. Judging from the rapid proliferation of hospital websites touting their ability to manage and intervene in TTTS cases and perhaps because of improved insurance coverage of fetal surgery for TTTS, there appeared a virtual arms race among hospitals to attract TTTS patients. Yet I required a hospital that permitted laser surgery for not only TTTS but also sIUGR. And I needed a doctor at that hospital who was experienced in conducting that unusual and controversial surgery.

What factors led to highest quality of care for TTTS and the survival of both twins?[1] For one, volume is determinative. The best TTTS outcomes, with mother and two babies alive and well after birth, are found at only those hospitals that have treated many TTTS cases. The other critical criterion is specialization. Hospitals specializing in TTTS employ the fetal therapists, neonatologists, obstetricians, ultrasound technicians, cardiologists, pediatricians, and the host of other medical professionals necessary to guide a TTTS pregnancy to a safe conclusion.

Perusing the flashy hospital websites, all with embedded oxymoronic video-clips of mothers telling sad tales of the survival of at least one twin, I identified only two US hospitals whose IRBs had approved laser surgery to treat combined TTTS and sIUGR cases: one was at a hospital in Miami, the other was at a hospital in Hollywood. I had friends in Los Angeles, and I called them to ask whether I could stay with them for a week or so—at an uncertain date. They, of course, agreed to host me. Although the Hollywood hospital would be more convenient now that I had housing there, I wondered which hospital had the more experienced doctors with combined TTTS and sIUGR. I then began working through the file of studies I'd collected on fetal surgery and TTTS. As a lawyer, I know to pay attention to studies' footnotes, where the real information for any argument or counterargument is located.

Jackpot: buried in a European study of fetal surgery on twins was a citation to a 2001 American study limited to twenty-eight sIUGR pregnancies in which laser ablation was used for eleven pregnancies to separate blood vessels that connected through the amnions.[2] This older American study, although limited, suggested that laser surgery reduced the risks of death of the larger fetus and neurological damage in newborn babies. There was no systematic neurological follow-up with the babies, however.[3]

This clue led me closer to my goal of having my difficult pregnancy end with the birth of at least one neurologically healthy child. The existence of a study about laser surgery for sIUGR twins meant someone was studying the issue—and that there was evidence to satisfy the next IRB review I would have to undergo. The lead author for the American twin study was the same doctor who had defined the five-step staging description for TTTS and had invented TTTS laser ablation surgery. He was located at the Miami TTTS-specialized hospital, which also permitted laser surgeries for sIUGR. I wrote him immediately:

Dear Dr. Q,

I hope you might be able to help me. I am 17.5 weeks pregnant with mono-di twins who are suspected of having TTTS and one of whom has sIUGR. My fetal medicine physician is Dr. Z. Unfortunately, Dr. Z cannot make a definitive TTTS diagnosis because the fluid level for the donor twin has not dropped below 2 cm, although Doppler studies show an absent diastolic flow to the donor and there is greater than 20% size difference between donor and recipient. sIUGR has been diagnosed based on greatly unequal placental share and the donor's two vessel umbilical cord and marginal cord insertion.

Without a TTTS diagnosis, Dr. Z says he is prohibited from doing a laser ablation procedure to coagulate connecting blood vessels in the fetuses' membranes. (I've checked with the FDA and am informed that there is no such prohibition from their perspective.) Dr. Z believes the only procedure available to address a sIUGR diagnosis is cord coagulation of the donor through the sac of the recipient using a 2mm rigid scope that would not permit good visualization of the amnions. Further complicating this scenario is that my placenta is mostly anterior with some fundal "wrap around."

Are you able and willing to do a laser ablation procedure to address sIUGR? I have read a European study that discusses this procedure, and I have also read your 2001 paper referenced at endnote 11.[4] I understand that there would be a poor prognosis for the donor if laser ablation were used, but I also understand there may be a better prognosis of a birth of a neurologically normal recipient than if cord coagulation is attempted with a non-flexible scope.

Time is now of the essence, for if I had to terminate the pregnancy because of grim prognosis for both twins, I would have to do so over the next two weeks. If you do perform laser ablations for patients like me, would you be able to see me in the upcoming week? I would be pleased to fly to Miami to meet with you.

> Thank you,
> GG

Doctor Q immediately returned my email, saying that there was no reason to choose cord coagulation for combined sIUGR and TTTS and that he could help me. He then called me the next day, a Saturday, and spoke with me for an hour about the potential of laser surgery to improve my pregnancy. He could not promise me any particular outcome but pointed out that he had been doing amniotic laser ablations for longer than anyone else and that he had trained most of the other surgeons at other hospitals that provided TTTS treatment. I agreed to fly to Miami that next week and to stay until he could perform my surgery. The doctor agreed to submit my case to his hospital's IRB and thought that its approval would be forthcoming very soon.

Now that I had found a hospital willing to permit an operation, I faced the reality that there was no guarantee of a positive outcome of fetal surgery. No one really knew what outcomes could be anticipated from laser ablation for sIUGR or for TTTS cases confounded by other complications. European studies of fetal surgery for sIUGR came to different conclusions than did American doctors who reviewed those studies. A 2007 to 2009 study from Belgium and Spain found that the full story for surgical care and management for TTTS and sIUGR could not be told solely from the standard assessment algorithms of fetal growth, amniotic fluid depth, and blood flow to the donor fetus.[5] The Europeans concluded that separating the twins' connecting blood vessels would protect the larger twin from the effects of hemorrhage in the event the smaller twin died from the effects of sIUGR.[6] The European study authors warned, though, that laser coagulation in sIUGR pregnancies is "technically difficult and not always feasible," and that separating the twins' connecting blood vessels would "significantly increase" the likelihood of the death of the smaller, growth-restricted fetus.[7] Not enough data were available for the European authors to conclude whether laser ablation of the twins' amnions would result in the larger twin's being born neurologically normal.

In contrast, a group of American doctors found that using laser surgery in sIUGR pregnancies did not improve the outcome for the larger twin and caused the likely demise of the smaller twin. Laser ablation of the connecting blood vessels virtually guaranteed the death of one twin in 70 percent of cases, and it had little effect on the number of physical and neurological problems that the larger sIUGR twin would suffer regardless of any intervention.[8] Therefore, said the Americans, the data did not indicate which of any interventions, including laser surgery, was the best course of action for sIUGR twins.[9] The Chinese weighed in as well. In a study published in early 2013, Chinese doctors found that doing nothing for sIUGR was not an option. The perinatal outcome of identical twins with sIUGR was "poor."[10] Both twins were at high risk of dying in utero.[11]

Each hospital IRB read these competing study conclusions to mean different things. Those hospitals with the lead American study authors on staff usually prohibited laser surgery for sIUGR. But hospitals with European study authors generally permitted this surgery. The hospital in Miami seemed to be an outlier, aligning itself with the European consensus that was more supportive of permitting expectant mothers to "maximize their chances at having one normal infant."[12] Laser ablation could be one of the tools available to these women and their doctors to manage sIUGR pregnancies.

Everyone—the Americans, Europeans, and Chinese—was waiting for the outcomes of a larger and longer-term Dutch twin study that would provide an answer to a key piece of the puzzle for managing TTTS and sIUGR: what could be done to avoid the 15 percent rate of neurological damage that afflicts babies with untreated sIUGR? Doctors in several European hospitals were conducting follow-up with over three hundred babies to compare the neurological health of those whose twin pregnancies had been managed with cord occlusion of the smaller twin with the outcomes of babies whose mothers had undergone laser ablation.[13] The hypothesis was that laser surgery intervention for sIUGR would protect the larger twin from the neurological consequences of the smaller twin's death while still giving the smaller twin a chance of survival. Final results from this study would not be available until the end of 2015 or 2016, too late to help me.

I prepared to fly to Miami, but then disaster struck. The Miami hospital's ethical review board withdrew its approval for laser surgery intervention in sIUGR cases. Dr. Q immediately resigned in protest. He called me in a fury to say that the hospital had kowtowed to the antiabortion movement and prohibited all fetal interventions that could result in the death of the fetus. He said that he would be moving to Belgium, where one teaching hospital continued to research sIUGR and combined sIUGR and TTTS interventions. The doctor invited me to follow him to Belgium, although it would take him a couple of weeks to set up shop there. He also cautioned that, possibly related to the scopes or surgical practices used, the outcomes in Europe of laser surgery were much worse than in the United States.

My pregnancy had advanced past eighteen weeks. It was too late to arrange for IRB approval and sIUGR surgery in Hollywood, and in any event, that hospital too stopped providing laser ablation for sIUGR soon after the hospital in Miami decided not to permit the procedure. Interestingly, hospitals in St. Louis[14] and in Seattle[15] later added laser surgery as options to treat sIUGR. The current websites for each brag that they are one of the only hospitals in the United States that will permit laser surgery for sIUGR.

My search for an intervention to save both twins from sIUGR had reached the end of the line. As for an intervention for TTTS, which also might be used to treat sIUGR as a complication of TTTS, I had a few more weeks to see whether the twins' amniotic fluid depths would meet the criteria for surgical intervention. The permissible timeline for TTTS surgeries had been extended to twenty-six weeks of gestation if I could find a doctor willing to operate this late in my pregnancy.[16]

My case had attracted attention from other doctors throughout the United States, several of whom were emailing and calling me regularly to monitor my prognosis. I responded to two of these doctors, from a hospital in Texas, with the following summary of my case:

Hello Dr. A and Dr. W,
Thank you very much for checking in with me.

I spoke to a contact at the FDA about the use of various scopes to conduct laser ablations in the case of sIUGR with absent or reverse flow. My contact at FDA put me in touch with the manufacturer of the particular scopes used for laser ablations, Storz, and provided me with a draft guidance document.[17]

As two FDA colleagues explained to me, the FDA does not regulate the practice of medicine and an exception could be obtained from Storz's marketing humanitarian device exemption (HDE) so that a laser ablation could be performed to address the sIUGR. However, an IRB determination would need to support this decision (see the draft guidance at question 29). Dr. Z was concerned about an adverse Hopkins IRB ruling that would, in effect, prevent him from doing laser surgery in my case. However, University of Miami, FL, and LA Children's Hospital permit their physicians to do laser ablations to address sIUGR with poor flow; in fact, neither of these locations offer cord occlusion for this problem.

In any event, I currently am not a candidate for any intervention, as my Dopplers and the fluid level of the donor fetus have improved slightly. As of yesterday, I'm 18.5 weeks, the fetuses have a 30% growth disparity, the recipient has around 9 cm fluid and the donor has about 2.85 cm, and the Dopplers generally show a positive diastolic flow. These measurements mean that I'm neither at TTTS nor have I reached a severe stage of sIUGR. The donor has a two-vessel cord with marginal insertion and a teeny, tiny bladder; but somehow, that fetus is still hanging in there. (Dr. X, with whom I talked yesterday, told me he is "shocked" that I am still pregnant; he's not the only one.)

But I'm advised to keep the pregnancy, as the chance of two neurologically healthy babies is high enough to warrant the risks. (And maternal discomfort: I look like the Goodyear blimp.) I hope you agree; if not, please do tell me!

Sincerely,

GG

The doctors tracking my pregnancy told me that I was at the very edge of science. No one knew what the interplay of TTTS and sIUGR, along with the cord and placental share issues faced by the smaller twin, could mean for the pregnancy or for long-term neurological outcomes of any babies born. My high-risk obstetrician said that I still had a fifty-fifty chance of developing the signs of full-blown TTTS, requiring me to have fetal laser surgery at some point during the nineteenth to twenty-sixth week of pregnancy. If that were to occur, I would return to Dr. Z at Hopkins for him to perform the laser ablation of the fetuses' blood vessels traveling through their membranes. If a Doppler showed blood flow from my placenta to the small fetus stopped completely or reversed in direction, I also could ask Dr. Z to perform a cord coagulation to try to save the larger twin. If the reverse blood flow were not detected immediately and a routine ultrasound showed clear brain or heart damage to the recipient, I would try to find a provider who would terminate the pregnancy.

My high-risk obstetrician conducted weekly ultrasounds to monitor the fluid levels in the twins' amniotic sacs and the blood flow to their hearts. Every week, the ultrasound tech selected a few of the clearest images of each twin, printed them, and handed the pictures to me on my way out the door. The ultrasound printouts were grainy, black-and-white Polaroids that spooled one after the other on a coated piece of paper, like a string of $3.00-off coupons from the neighborhood pharmacy. Most parents treasure these first photos of their children, posting them on Facebook and proudly displaying them in their offices. Ultrasound photos are routinely shown off at baby showers and sent to the grandparents. But not mine. I trashed them as soon as I got home.

The pictures depressed me, for they constructed a progressive, visual story of how poorly my pregnancy was going. If everything went south, as I was convinced it soon would, I did not want photographs to remind me of how bad it all had been. Not a single ultrasound picture remains of my twins.

Before obstetrical ultrasounds became routine, beginning in the late 1970s, what occurred during a pregnancy was optically unknowable, with the uterus as a black box. Now, visit by visit and frame by frame, a pregnancy can be documented from start to finish. Sonograms are the standard of care for all pregnancies because they show how the pregnancy is developing. For pregnancies with multiples, ultrasounds are critical for diagnosing TTTS and sIUGR, among other complications, and providing guidance as to how to resolve these problems.

Beyond serving as obstetrical tools, ultrasound images have been weaponized in the war against abortion. Activists seeking to curtail abortions credit sonogram photos for changing women's minds about terminating their pregnancies.[18] If these photos are the first baby pictures, then the images they show must be of babies, not merely of clumps of cells or developing fetuses. The presumption is that viewing an ultrasound picture of her pregnancy will have such an emotional effect on a woman that, wracked with guilt, she will be unable to carry through with her planned abortion.

Policymakers have seized on the belief that ultrasound images are baby pictures and the assumption that women are fickle and easily persuaded to become mothers. Eighteen states have passed laws that require abortion providers to offer women an opportunity to view an ultrasound image of their pregnancy before its termination, and five states mandate that the woman actually gaze at the image. In some states, Oklahoma, for example, the physician must verbally describe the ultrasound in detail to the woman. For pregnancies too early to be depicted with standard ultrasound, the provider must insert a wand in the woman's vagina to capture the image. Alabama requires women to sign an affidavit if they refuse to look at the sonogram.[19] If the woman nevertheless persisted in her obstinate desire for an abortion, proposed federal laws would stop her. At the writing of this book, currently pending before the US House of Representatives is the Heartbeat Protection Act of 2021, which would prohibit physicians from aborting a fetus that has a heartbeat detectable by "standard medical practice."[20] Criminal penalties of a fine, up to five years in prison, or both would punish any doctor who went forward with an abortion after a heartbeat is detected, even for fetuses with fatal abnormalities or conditions and for mothers with psychological or emotional conditions.

Ironically, women seeking an abortion may not be dissuaded by being forced to view an ultrasound image. It turns out that women know exactly what they are doing and, if at an abortion clinic, are well aware that they are pregnant. They also understand that pregnancy results in babies. But women may have a myriad of reasons for choosing to end a pregnancy, and viewing an ultrasound of the pregnancy does not vitiate a woman's resolve in going forward with an abortion.[21] Forced ultrasounds for abortion patients negatively affects only their rights to autonomy, privacy, and unimpeded access to healthcare, not the abortion rate.[22]

Had the fetuses been stable and growing, my obstetrician forecast that I would be induced to give birth at thirty-six weeks and that the babies would emerge healthy and hale after spending some time in the neonatal intensive care unit (NICU). But the smaller twin was not doing well and was barely growing. Without enough blood from the placenta, his development had ground almost to a halt. More positively, the larger recipient twin was developing normally, yet his situation continued to be perilous. The ever-present risk for the larger fetus was that the donor twin would die, causing the recipient's blood pressure to drop and for him to hemorrhage and perish as well.

Another shoe dropped from this millipede of a pregnancy. Both fetuses' hearts now had defects that were visible in their ultrasounds and echocardiograms. Cardiovascular complications are common in TTTS. As my doctor described it, one baby's heart overworks and the other baby's heart grows lazy because its twin beats for two. Recipient twins suffer from heart problems affecting their cardiac function and pressure, even at early stages of TTTS.[23] Approximately 4 percent of recipient twins are born with an obstruction of their heart's right ventricle outflow tract. The donor twin too has health problems resulting from the reduced return blood flow the donor receives. Donor twins have an increased risk for a kink in their aorta, called aortic coarctation, putting still additional strain on their overtaxed hearts.[24] Strained hearts mean heart attacks, which would bring down both twins. They portend impeded development, which meant even slower growth for the donor twin. They may require fetal or neonatal open-heart surgery to correct. I added a cardiologist to the mix of doctors monitoring my care. By February that year, I had already exceeded my annual out-of-pocket maximum for my health insurance plan, and my employer had added me to a catastrophic care scheme. The expense of fetal cardiac care would be repaid somehow.

The twins were a costly losing battle, and I had gotten lost in the fog of war, trying every possible measure to save something that might not have been worth saving. My maternal-fetal specialist's office was located on the grounds of a Catholic hospital. After one visit, the doctor pulled me into the hallway and whispered that I might wish to terminate the entire pregnancy. Hospital policy, which was based on the Catholic Church's prohibition of abortion for any reason, prohibited him from discussing this option with me. His medical ethics demanded that he help me, though, and he could see that I was suffering. He explained that a late-term abortion facility, one of the few left in the country, was located fifty miles away and that he could help me make an appointment there. He knew the clinic's doctor, who was a kind and compassionate man. But I would encounter protesters around the clinic, and I should be prepared to see and pass by them. Should he make the call to the abortion clinic?

Only 1 percent of abortions, or around fifteen thousand abortions per year in the United States, occur after twenty weeks of gestation.[25] This timing, although later in the pregnancy, is still before the fetus is viable. In medicine, viability is defined as the gestational age at which the chance of survival is 50 percent: around 23 to 24 weeks in developed countries and around 34 weeks in developing countries.[26] Once a fetus is viable, an abortion cannot happen; a preterm birth would.[27] The United States Supreme Court declared in the 1973 *Roe v. Wade* decision that abortion is a woman's fundamental right before the fetus's ability to survive outside its mother. After the fetus could be viable, the Supreme Court permits each state to regulate when and how an abortion could be procured.[28] States must permit abortions regardless of the gestational age of the fetus to preserve the life or health of the pregnant person.[29]

Forty-three states now set limits on when an abortion can be obtained, and most of these limits are based on calendar time but not on a particular fetus's projected viability, as required by *Roe v. Wade*.[30] Seventeen states have been successful in enacting abortion bans at twenty weeks after an estimated conception.[31] These bans are based on the erroneous belief that fetuses can feel pain after twenty weeks of development and that an abortion would be painful to the fetus.[32]

Some states' abortion laws violate the *Roe v. Wade* decision but have not been challenged in court. For example, Michigan permits a postviability abortion only if the mother's life is endangered by the pregnancy. This ban violates *Roe*'s requirement that an abortion be permitted if necessary to preserve the woman's health.[33] Other states parse the difference between a pregnant woman's mental health and her physical health, with most states permitting a health exception to a ban on late-term abortions only when the pregnancy endangers the mother's physical health.[34] Even if pregnancy has made the woman depressed, suicidal, or psychotic, these deleterious mental health conditions are not enough to warrant terminating the pregnancy.

I wonder what I would have done had I lived in Michigan or in any of the states that ban abortion after twenty weeks. My twins were far too small and undeveloped at twenty-one weeks to have survived, although it is possible that the larger one might have been considered viable and the smaller one not. Yet their circulatory systems were connected, so the viability of each depended on the other. My life was not at imminent risk in carrying them, but my life and health could have been endangered by the hemorrhaging of one of the fetuses or if I became hypertensive from the ballooning amniotic sac of the recipient fetus. It is obvious that state abortion bans were not written with consideration or empathy for situations like mine.

States' abortion bans have limited second- and third-trimester abortion providers to a tiny handful of locations with less restrictive laws.[35] In 2009, a Kansas doctor who provided abortions in the final months of pregnancy was murdered in his church. With that physician's death, only four late-term abortion doctors were left in the United States.[36] These doctors fly in and out the states where it remains legal for them to terminate the pregnancies that no other medical provider is willing or able to. The late-term abortion providers are older men who will want to retire from their arduous work. With state prohibitions on teaching abortion techniques to medical students, there might not be younger doctors to take their place. Soon in the United States, there may be nowhere to obtain pregnancy terminations between twenty and twenty-eight weeks of gestation.

The late-term abortion clinic in southern Maryland was surrounded constantly by protesters who were bussed in daily by their churches or parochial schools.[37] I knew their tactics well. On designated Saturdays and holidays when I was growing up, my family would occasionally stop by the women's clinic in our city to join the abortion protests. Vigorous protesting in inadequate shoes caused my mom to strain her feet. She limped around piteously and needed months of physical therapy and specially made orthotic inserts.

Annually, my Catholic high school provided a winter semester exam exemption to any student who went to Washington, DC, to join the *Roe v. Wade* protests in January. This is where my parents drew the line between support for Church teaching and devotion to good childrearing: I was absolutely prohibited from skipping my exams and joining the adolescent horde in the nation's capital. After driving overnight to DC in a yellow school bus, thousands of Catholic high schoolers were bunked like sardines on the gymnasium floor of the Catholic University of America. After more nights of no sleep because of hormonal mass make-out sessions with juvenile delinquents from across the country, the students were roused at dawn to march for twelve hours in sleet and subfreezing temperatures. Being teenagers, they refused to wear their coats and marched while clad only jeans and school sweatshirts. Each year, half the school returned with mononucleosis.

At the late-term abortion clinic in Maryland, around fifty people, many of whom were children, would stand on the sidewalk in front of the clinic with posters on sticks. From afar, they appeared a phalanx of soldiers with pikes of undulating, oversized placards picturing dismembered fetuses. These photographs are ostensibly the results of a late-term abortion, but their provenance is in doubt, as is the consent of the patient to have her abortion photographed.[38] The protesters would chant and sing, and when a woman approached the clinic, they would surge around her. They would shout at presumed patients, begging them not to abort and asking them why they wanted to kill their babies. Should a patient falter or slow her pace toward the clinic, the protesters would take this as a sign that their entreaties were having an effect. Their prayers would escalate in fervor and volume, and they would shout promises that they could assist the patient at their crisis pregnancy center down the street. They could show her an ultrasound that demonstrated that her fetus was alive and a wholly formed and separate child.

Of course, had they found themselves or their daughters in my situation, these abortion protesters would have become abortion patients in the very clinic they rallied outside.[39] For all their religiosity, the protesters could not work miracles, and their prayers alone would not change biology or embryology. Not one protester knew how to treat a fetus's congenital heart defects or a woman's depression at carrying a dying baby. And the protesters certainly did not know how to split apart blood vessels connecting through the amniotic membranes or how to improve the placental blood flow to a fetus that has stopped growing. They were no more capable than all maternal-fetal doctors in the United States in telling me whether laser surgery or cord occlusion would give me any hope of having one mentally and physically healthy child or whether both were exercises in futility.

As I considered for the millionth time whether to continue with my pregnancy or to terminate it, I telephoned an old friend, one who had worked with me on reproductive rights advocacy. I gave her a brief outline of how challenging my pregnancy had been and about the poor prognosis for my twins. I explained that aborting the pregnancy was on the table, but because the data and advice I had received was unclear about a preferred course of action, I had waited too long to decide what to do. My options for abortion were limited to the one nearby late-term clinic. After listening to me carefully for my entire sad soliloquy, my friend responded, simply, "I'll go with you to get the abortion. And I'll walk with you through the protesters." Her words remain the kindest I have ever heard.

After considering my options and what I would experience if I sought an abortion, I decided to keep the pregnancy, in the hope that one of the fetuses would be born unscathed. With my family and my years of indoctrination in Catholic school, an abortion this late in the pregnancy was a bridge too far, even if it would have been the most sensible resolution to my predicament. Given the poor prognosis for the smaller twin, my obstetrician told me that a premature birth was more likely to save the larger twin.

In preparation for my impending preterm birth, my doctor twice used an elephant-sized needle to shoot painful steroids into my butt to strengthen the fetuses' lungs and to speed their development. These injections of betamethasone are given twenty-four hours apart and are most effective for the first week after administration. If the patient does not go into labor within a week of the injections, a "rescue course" of more shots is sometimes given. But rescue courses of betamethasone are controversial for twins because there are no good studies that show their effectiveness.[40]

Birth is painted as if it were always a successful outcome of pregnancy, its goal. The outcomes for premature babies, those born before thirty-seven full weeks or whose weight and development is less than an average thirty-seven-week-old fetus, tell a different story. The earlier in its gestation a baby is born, the less likely its survival. The baby's heart may not be formed enough to pump blood or its lungs strong enough to breathe oxygen. The survival outcomes for boys are worse than those for girls.[41] Because almost half of twins deliver preterm, they have a postdelivery death rate that is seven times higher than that of singletons.[42] For babies extremely preterm that are born before 28 weeks or weigh fewer than a thousand grams, only about a third to half survive, and a fifth to half of the survivors are very sick.[43] More live if born very preterm at 28 to 32 weeks or moderately preterm at 32 to 34 weeks, but still, these babies are 60 percent of all infant deaths.[44] Less grim are the outcomes for late preterm babies born from 34 to less than 37 weeks. In well-resourced countries with good neonatal intensive care facilities, virtually all (99 percent) of these late preterm babies survive, but many nevertheless face a lifetime of health complications.[45]

Heavier premature babies have a better prognosis than do low birthweight babies, with survival improving dramatically for each hundred-gram increase in the baby's weight.[46] Weight is a protective factor for infants, indicating more complete development. A greater weight usually means the baby has a store of fat to sustain it until it can process food and to warm it, helping the baby to maintain its temperature.

I was justified in my worries about the expected survival for babies like mine, same-sex twins born at highly discordant weights. Surprisingly, if they survive immediately after birth, preemie twins tend to do better than premature singletons. But twin babies that have suffered from growth restriction, when one weighs much more than the other, have worse survival rates than single premature babies, especially if born extremely[47] or even moderately preterm.[48] Twins born before thirty-five weeks have significantly higher rates of death and illness than those permitted to gestate until they are full-term or at least thirty-seven weeks.[49]

If a premature baby lives and survives the immediate aftereffects of its birth, the baby likely will still struggle with sickness and the adverse consequences of being born too soon. Up to 10 percent of babies born prematurely and at low birth weight (below 1,500 grams) will develop mental retardation, visual disabilities, or neurological dysfunction.[50] Depending on the extent of its prematurity, the baby is likely to suffer from respiratory distress caused by underdeveloped lungs. Failure to provide the baby with oxygen immediately at its birth may cause the baby neurological damage. But using high-pressure respirators to force air into the baby's lungs may damage the baby's eyes, causing retinopathy of prematurity.

Many of these conditions require surgical intervention for babies who are only days old. For babies whose bowels are obstructed and necrotizing from a stomach and intestines that cannot tolerate even breast milk, abdominal surgery must be immediately provided. The baby may have brain bleeds from still-forming blood vessels, necessitating surgical implantation of shunts to release the pressure of the blood on the brain. Even late premature babies, ones that have made it to 36 weeks, will often require surgical fixes for inguinal hernias that result from a urogenital tract that develops fully only from 36 to 40 weeks.

A parent's greatest fear of giving birth prematurely is that her baby's quality of life may be forever compromised. Prematurity is associated with learning and motor disabilities and with visual and hearing impairment, contributing to approximately half the disabilities in children.[51] After all the effort I had made to protect my fetuses from neurological damage, I was sobered by the likelihood of a premature birth's causing the twins cerebral palsy or cognitive delay. All premature babies have a significant risk, over 5 percent,[52] of developing cerebral palsy. This permanent neurological impairment is usually the result of brain damage to the baby before or during birth. Cerebral palsy may prevent the child from speaking, walking, talking, controlling its body, or living independently. Alternatively, even if it does not have cerebral palsy, the child may also have cognitive disabilities that prevent intellectual development. Risk of cerebral palsy and cognitive impairment is associated with the extent of prematurity of the baby, with a 6.1 percent risk of cerebral palsy and over a 7 percent risk of cognitive delay for babies born at or before 28 weeks.[53] There is a 2.4 percent risk of cerebral palsy for babies born between

32 to 34 gestational weeks, and about a half a percent risk for preemies born after 34 weeks.[54] Even for babies not considered premature, who are born early term at 37 or 38 weeks, the risk of cerebral palsy is almost doubled compared to that for full-term babies.[55]

The considerable concerns related to premature birth notwithstanding, I was vexed that my doctors seemed to presume that they should induce me to deliver the twins prematurely. They argued that there was "deterioration" at thirty-six weeks for twins, but this belief was based on no scientific data I could find. Back to my Google searches, which quickly confirmed the absence of evidence that twins should gestate any less than a single baby. A group of authors in the scientific journal *Nature* noted the dearth of support for inducing premature delivery for twins before thirty-seven weeks, writing that "there are no data to support discretionary preterm birth."[56]

I was ready to march into my obstetrician's office, waving the *Nature* article aloft and preparing for war to stop any induction of a preterm birth. A midwife friend told me to hold my fire. She explained that deterioration usually refers to the mother and not the baby. Later in the pregnancy, when exactly is unknown, the placenta stops functioning as well as it had been. Blood stops moving through the umbilical cord, causing the fetus to stop developing. In response, the physicians institute close monitoring of the blood flow from the placenta to the fetus and measure the fetus's continued growth. If problems are detected, labor might be induced; or if the baby's results are very concerning and require an immediate birth, a caesarean section may be warranted.

My doctor was now conducting twice-weekly ultrasounds to determine the blood flow to the twins and their growth, so I was not worried that my deteriorating placenta would somehow be missed. My greater preoccupation was avoiding at all costs the grave and certain risks of prematurity. Even if it was backed only by anecdote, not by any known study, the presumption was that a twin mother's placenta would give up the ghost somewhere between thirty-six and thirty-eight weeks. I would aim to go into labor or be induced during this window. It would net my twins almost a full-term pregnancy and was beyond the timing of the most severe neurological and physical repercussions of a premature birth.

Chapter Eight

Snake Oil and Doulas

My cervix was thinned, or effaced, and its length shrank constantly. Soon, I would no longer be able to hold in the twins, and I would be in preterm labor. My doctor ordered me to reduce pressure on my cervix, so I started asking to sit on my forty-five-minute-long morning and afternoon commute by train. Twice, those occupying the seats declined my request, with one fellow telling me, "I got here first." Fair enough, but there were many folks seated around him. Everyone else feigned deafness and blindness to prevent them from having to relinquish their seats to the pregnant-with-twins woman. In frustration, my doctor ordered me to bed, despite the evidence that bed rest does nothing to improve outcomes in twin pregnancies and may harm the mother.

Little is known about what will improve the outcome of twin pregnancies; snake oil may be as effective as bed rest, cerclage, and tocolytics, which successfully ward off preterm birth for singletons.[1] A meta-analysis of seven trials involving 713 women and 1,452 babies found that bed rest is futile for women pregnant with multiples.[2] Hospitalizing a twin mom to force her to rest did reduce the outcome of premature birth for the babies. But resting at home has not been well studied for women with multiples. Bed rest possibly and perversely might make things worse, with some studies finding preterm birth increased for women on bed rest.[3]

Bed rest also is depressing, with the woman confined to her room—or to a hospital bed, for those in immediate danger of premature rupture of their amniotic sacs—in terror that her inadvertent movement might harm her developing fetuses. Conducted properly, bed rest can harm you, even as it gives your fetuses a better chance of survival. Women able to follow their doctors' orders to reduce all movement may develop blood clots and bone thinning.

Realistically, few can cease all activity and rest in bed. For women with young children or inflexible work schedules, bed rest is an impossibility. Growing new babies doesn't mean the current ones stop requiring food or diaper changes. From the time he turned two, my first child had to learn to walk everywhere and to crawl into his own car seat; I could no longer carry him. But he still needed care, cuddles, and active, not bedbound, supervision. My job did not permit telecommuting and would have required me to take unpaid leave if I was officially on bed rest. Luckily for me, my supervisor turned a blind eye to my routine absence in my cubicle, noting to anyone who inquired that my work continued to be completed.

Cerclage is stitching a woman's cervix shut so that a baby cannot emerge from it prematurely. A normal person pregnant with twins has a cervix that is around 50 millimeters at the beginning of her pregnancy and around 30 millimeters long by the third trimester.[4] A cervix of less than 30 millimeters long spells trouble for the pregnancy: the shorter the cervix, the greater the likelihood of a preterm birth.[5] If the cervix is dangerously short, less than 15 millimeters, or is dilated, a premature birth is almost certain. My cervical length was less than 20 millimeters and nosediving. Doctors will offer cerclage to a woman pregnant with a single baby and with a shortened cervix. For twins, though, this intervention was an exercise in futility, with no evidence that cerclage prevented preterm birth.[6] In twin pregnancies, cerclage had been studied in a dedicated randomized controlled trial only once and in 1982.[7] That study suggested that, like bed rest, cerclage might expose the woman to harm. Cerclage could cause infections, making it twice as likely that a woman will deliver her twins before thirty-five weeks.

Tocolytics, drugs to stave off preterm labor, are also routinely prescribed for women pregnant with twins, again with no or worsening effect. Nifedipine and indomethacin tocolysis for women in preterm labor may delay delivery for between two and three days for pregnancies of more than twenty-six weeks.[8] In other words, even with the medicine, women deliver prematurely. A mother's taking tocolytics does nothing to help her twin babies, who still die and suffer neonatal complications at equal rates to those twins whose mothers did not use the meds.[9] However, tocolytics use imperils the health of twin moms, placing them at risk for pulmonary edema and increasing the risk that the mother herself will die before she can deliver her twins.[10]

The TTTS Foundation website, which dates from 1989 and, after decades of stagnation, was updated at the beginning of 2021, advises pregnant women to consume high levels of protein.[11] No studies are referenced, and no data are given about the efficacy of chugging protein shakes, but anecdotes from one doctor are presented as facts.[12] Nevertheless, the website guilts mothers into drinking as much protein as they can consume: "Mothers also feel immediate satisfaction knowing that there is something they can do right away to help their babies."

Even with a master's degree in public health, I fell for the hype and to the guilt. Why wouldn't I do everything possible to help my babies? Ignoring the five hundred calories per drink, I downed protein shakes several times a day and promptly gained fifty pounds. I rested with my feet in the air and did not pick up my toddler, even when he cried. I took maternity leave early, against company policy. I took pills to stave off labor for one day more.

The tocolytics and the bed rest were so discombobulating that I accidently purchased a new home—in a different state from the one I lived in. Adding two more children meant we would morph from a family of three to a family of five, but my spouse's house, which he had owned for decades as a bachelor, had only two bedrooms. We had held off looking for a replacement home until we knew whether we would be adding no, one, or two children to our family. By the time it was evident the pregnancy would stick, we were almost out of time. We put in bids on every larger house for sale in our Maryland neighborhood, and, in the fevered, real estate market, we were outbid on all of them. Giving up, we hired an architect to draw up plans to remodel the house we were in, telling ourselves that our two newborns, our toddler, and the two of us could stay in a hotel for a couple of weeks while the construction was taking place. We were raving mad.

One pretty Saturday in May, we were seduced by the flowering azaleas, went out for a drive, and passed an open house about a mile from our current one. Stopping in, I was wowed by the staging: walls and ceilings painted in various shades of taupe, white furniture, and glass tables spread across what seemed acres of an open floor plan. I spent more time checking out the hand stitching on a Turkish floor rug than noting how many bedrooms or baths the house had. We put in a bid for the place and two others we had seen and promptly forgot about it, both of us being very busy and distracted. My spouse had a major court case, and I was trying not to go into premature labor. When our realtor called later to congratulate us on buying "the DC house," we were both crashed out on separate couches in our tiny living room. We looked at each other and said in unison, "What DC house?!" Of the house's many features and attributes we had overlooked, the most significant was that it was on the District of Columbia side of a street that was split between DC and Maryland. An interstate move would mean new taxes, changed drivers' licenses, different laws applicable to employing our nanny, revised bar admission requirements for practicing as attorneys, and a less desirable school district. But we were stuck. Our offer had been accepted and our sizeable earnest money check had been cashed.

From my bed, where I was supposed to be resting, I completed the home purchase and move from my iPhone. I electronically signed onto a mortgage with my spouse, obligating us to one another at a tune of hundreds of thousands of dollars. I hired movers online through Task Rabbit and bought furniture on Craigslist. I perused paint chips on my computer and because what appears on a screen looks nothing at all like what will be on a wall, selected hideous, clashing colors. The painters, whom I also found on the internet, followed my instructions to paint the bedrooms mustard yellow and neon orange. Instead of jewel-toned elegance in coral and gold, the upstairs resembles a Texas barbecue. In a brief stint of nesting, until my doctor found out and prohibited it, I climbed ladders and attempted to hang curtains. We closed on the sale of our old house and moved into the new one four days before I gave birth.

An accidental, cross-jurisdictional home purchase was a clear indication that, in addition to my complicated pregnancy, I was suffering from another malady: mommy brain.[13] For pregnant women and new mothers, the act of thinking feels as if their brains are sloshing through sticky swamp mud during a foggy night. Their reactions are slow, their mental acuity reduced, and their ability to name people or . . . that something or other, nonexistent. Scientists claim that no convincing evidence exists that pregnancy causes an overall decline in cognitive performance or memory.[14] Studies conducted pre- and postpregnancy found "no loss of memory, verbal skills, or working memory."[15] Ever the randomized controlled trial adherent, I nevertheless call bullshit. Perhaps it was the hormones or the sleep deprivation or the crushing, constant, worrisome preoccupation with dying while creating life, but I was dumb when I used to be smart. Other women report the same.

One hypothesis is that a human can do only so much. Unable, metaphorically, to pat her head while rubbing her stomach or to walk and chew gum at the same time, a woman's body must allocate its resources between the competing energy requirements of the mother's brain and the developing fetus.[16] The fetus wins this struggle, leading to a decline in maternal cognition during gestation.

The science is unstable, though. There is wide agreement that pregnancy changes a woman's brain, but studies are contradictory about what changes, when, and the effects of this change. Some say maternal gray matter increases, others find a decrease, and still others indicate that changes occur in other regions of the brain. The nature and magnitude of pregnancy-related neural adaptations may be contingent on the specific time window during which they are measured.[17] And "maternal cognition" is multivariate, with declines in some areas leading to enhancements in others. Brains are flexible and elastic, constantly modifying themselves in response to new life experiences and learning. Head space real estate is limited, so the brain dispenses with whatever is not required and adds onto areas that are. To make up for any loss of gray matter, the brain's hippocampus expands after pregnancy.[18]

Pregnant women may, as a result, be impaired in their ability to remember words, but they experience improved social cognition, including in empathetic understanding.[19] The pregnant brain's bolstering of areas involved in perceiving the feelings and perspectives of others might be a necessary adaptation allowing a mother's bonding with her infant.[20] Too little brain change could be associated with poor ability to provide the concentrated care required for infant survival.[21] Pregnancy-caused brain transformations, just like those in the breasts, pelvis, and blood volume, are those that make a woman into a mother.[22]

Just as postpartum childcare lasts for decades, mommy brain's effects are equally long-lasting. One study found brain changes two years after pregnancy,[23] and another traced vestiges of them even decades after childbirth.[24] Interestingly, pregnancy's brain fog effect is supposed to be short-lived, and pregnancy has a long-term and beneficial consequence on maternal brain health. A higher number of previous childbirths is associated with less apparent brain aging, with mothers having lower brain inflammation and related disease during their childbearing years and beyond into old age.[25]

For me, the brain changes of childbearing are not the rosy side effects that science paints them to be. My pregnant season has long passed, but in writing this book, I've penned this chapter at least twice. Or I think I have. The studies on mommy brain are very familiar to me, and I am certain these paragraphs have been drafted before. But I cannot find my earlier research anywhere, even as I sort through the multiple versions of this work on two laptops, two Dropboxes, and a One Drive. Pieces of my writing have disappeared into the ether, like lost socks and gloves and one of every pair of baby shoes. And, likely, my sanity itself.

In my haze of confusion, I needed to locate a hospital that had both a labor and delivery ward for me and a high-level NICU for the twins. The babies were the priority, with my desired birth experience a distant afterthought. Having a birth center birth, as I had done with my first baby and would greatly have preferred for my own privacy and comfort, was completely out of the question. DC has only one freestanding birth center staffed by midwives, and that facility does not accept patients gestating twins. It also cannot assume the liability of assisting the birth of medically compromised, premature infants.[26]

Nor could I just go to the nearest hospital whenever I went into labor. Provided they passed thirty-two weeks, when the smallest, donor twin would be viable, whether both twins survived would depend on where they were born and the adequacy of care they received at that location. Few hospitals would be up to the task; it was incumbent on me, the mother, to determine what setting would have the right mix of skilled doctors, equipment, and policy to ensure the best outcome for me and my twins. In addition, the hospital had to be an easy commute from my home, given that a lengthy NICU stay was likely for the babies and that I would be shuttling back and forth, caring for my first, second, and third children.

The never-ending need to decide made my pregnancy exhausting. I could not put everything on autopilot and trust it would all turn out for the best. Instead, I could never give up the fight. Overwhelmingly, I felt the pregnancy was mine to save and mine to lose if I made the wrong decisions. Door A, we all come out alive; Door B, two of us; Door C, one survivor; Door D, no one. What blame would I bear if, failing to read the most current article or to ask the right question, my twins perished? After all, it is always the mother's fault.

Newborn hospital care facilities are rated in order of specialty from Level 1 to Level 4.[27] Babies can be transported by ambulance or helicopter from one level of care to another, going up or down a level according to their needs. To avoid the horror of a cross-town or cross-state transfer of a fragile newborn, the mother is advised to anticipate the level of NICU that will be required and to try to give birth at the same hospital as where that NICU is located. She is to control a process over which she has no control. The first NICU levels, 1 and 2, are not intensive care facilities at all but rather are nurseries. A Level 1 is for well newborns with providers equipped to care for healthy, stable babies who were born at term at around 40 weeks. Sick or premature babies are moved elsewhere. A Level 2 special care nursery can provide medical attention to babies born at or after 32 weeks who weigh more than 1,500 grams (3.3 pounds). Level 2s also can house babies who have just been discharged from a Level 3 or higher NICU and are growing and doing well. Babies requiring ventilators to help them breathe, born before 32 weeks, or weighing less than 1,500 grams must be moved to a higher level of care.

For TTTS/sIUGR babies who are likely to be born prematurely and at low weights, a Level 1 or 2 nursery is a terrible idea. Studies show survival improvement rates of more than 300 percent when fragile babies are born at NICUs that are Level 3 and higher.[28] As with CVS, amniocentesis, laser surgery for TTTS, and ultrasound interpretation for sIUGR, volume also is critical. You do not want to be the first TTTS pregnancy a hospital has seen and its test case. Neonatal survival is markedly better in NICUs with experience of caring for more than fifty premature newborns annually.[29]

This brings us to a Level 3, a true neonatal intensive care unit. A Level 3 has a clinical team able to care for tiny babies weighing less than 1,500 grams or those born before thirty-two weeks. It also has the equipment needed to help babies breathe and pediatric providers specialized in treating infants' hearts, lungs, and kidneys. The one thing a Level 3 cannot do is surgery, but it is the minimum level NICU appropriate for newborns with the effects of TTTS and sIUGR.

A Level 4 NICU offers the highest level of care for newborns and is the regional receiving hospital for babies transported there from lower level nurseries. A Level 4 can operate on babies who have birth defects, including heart conditions. It also is equipped with the personnel and machines to care for very sick babies. In classic grade creep, certain Level 4 NICUs hold themselves out as Level 5. The only difference between a Level 4 and a Level 5 NICU is, as it was explained to me, the helipad. If a baby can be transported to a NICU by helicopter and land on the facility's roof, that's a Level 5.

A team of pediatric specialists, including pediatric anesthesiologists and ophthalmologists, would be required to help the twins survive. Because heart or neurological surgery might be required for the twins, my preference was for a Level 4 NICU, which would have pediatric surgical specialists onsite. And because I, like all mothers, wanted what I perceived as "the best" for my babies and because helicopters are cool, I tried to find a Level 5 NICU, helipad and all.

What the hospital could do for my twins was important, but so too was what the hospital would *not* do. In addition to having a high-level NICU, skilled labor and delivery ward, and convenient location, the hospital also needed to have a policy of nonresuscitation. If one or both twins was born too tiny to survive without significant—and likely debilitating—intervention, I sought a hospital that would follow my wishes about aggressive resuscitation of my newborn twins. Specifically, I wanted assurance that the hospital would not automatically resuscitate either twin if he were born very early, very small, or in a very compromised condition. I wanted to be the one who would determine whether resuscitation would be offered to my own babies.

One out of ten babies born will require simple stimulation, drying, light rubbing, and repositioning at birth to help them breathe. Of these, 3 to 6 percent need "basic" resuscitation with a hand-operated bag and facemask. I had no concerns whatsoever with the use of these modest measures, which are used in even the most resource-poor settings. My objections were to "advanced" resuscitation offered to less than 1 percent of babies, approximately 1.4 million per year, primarily in wealthy countries. These advanced measures include intubation for positive pressure mechanical ventilation.[30] Advanced measures save newborns' lives, especially babies born very prematurely. Data published for newborns delivered in the United States, England, and Australia within the past decade have indicated rates of survival of about a quarter for births at 23 weeks, about a half for births at 24 weeks, and between two-thirds and three-quarters for births at 25 weeks of gestation.[31] Survival comes at a cost, however. In the United States, only one-third of infants born at 24 weeks lived without significant neurological impairment, defined as cerebral palsy, blindness, profound hearing loss, or intellectual developmental two standard deviations or more below the mean.[32]

These harms are sometimes caused by the resuscitation methods used on the babies. Intubation and mechanical ventilation frequently result in bronchopulmonary dysplasia, leading to chronic lung disease persisting into adulthood. Babies who were on machine ventilators had "increased susceptibility to respiratory infections, asthma, pulmonary hypertension, frequent hospital admissions, neurodevelopmental delays, and higher mortality."[33] Over the course of ten years, extreme measures in neonatal resuscitation obtained a miniscule, absolute change of only 4 percent in premature babies' survival without impairment.[34] Adverse outcomes of advanced resuscitation, including significant neurodevelopmental impairment, remain stagnant.[35]

The American Academy of Pediatrics (AAP) guidelines on neonatal resuscitation, which reflect the poor survival and health outcomes for very premature babies, say that resuscitation should be obligatory beginning at 25 weeks' gestation, optional at 24 weeks, and unusual at 23 weeks.[36] Gestational age provides the only guidance for doctors to determine when or how to resuscitate; no advice is given regarding infants with conditions such as TTTS and sIUGR and who have poor development despite their gestational age.[37] And a baby's survival at discharge from the NICU does not improve a doctor's ability to estimate the child's likelihood of survival through the first 18 to 22 months after birth.[38] Ultimately, the AAP punts decisions about appropriateness of resuscitation before 25 weeks of gestation to region-specific guidelines.[39]

That's an incredibly challenging problem. Whereas in other countries, such as the Netherlands and Switzerland, there are not policies or community consensus supporting aggressive treatment for babies born at very early gestational ages (leading to a high mortality rate for micropreemies),[40] in the United States resuscitation policy varies state by state and hospital by hospital, with enormous variation among them.[41] American doctors and hospital administrators are not in uniform agreement about when they should defer to parents' wishes about the care of their newborn child. "Reasonable international consensus exists among bioethicists that between 23 weeks and 0 days, and 24 weeks and 6 days, resuscitation may be provided or may be withheld" according to the parents' wishes.[42] When, as there is with premature birth, there is genuine uncertainty and the outcome could be either a healthy life or terrible death, hospital staff should not overrule parental decisions about the care of their infants.[43]

Reasonableness and reality seldom meet in the United States, however. A 2003 Texas Supreme Court case, *Miller v. HCA*, found in favor of a neonatologist who resuscitated a severely premature infant against the wishes of the parents. The child survived, although, at seven years old, she "could not walk, talk, feed herself, or sit up on her own. . . . [She] was legally blind, suffered from mental retardation, cerebral palsy, seizures, and spastic quadriparesis in her limbs. She could not be toilet-trained and required a shunt in her brain to drain fluids that accumulate there and needed care twenty-four hours a day. The evidence further demonstrated that her circumstances will not change."[44] This permanent and ongoing harm notwithstanding, according to the ruling, physicians who are faced with split-second, life-or-death decisions do not need parental consent to provide life-sustaining treatment to minors.[45] The court's decision remains good law in Texas and had for decades a chilling effect on respect for parental decision-making in the rest of the United States, where "years of legal wrangling are a norm."[46]

At least the pregnant patient could anticipate the reception she would receive at a Catholic hospital if she requested withholding of resuscitation from her severely compromised newborn. Catholic hospitals apply their religious doctrine, as expressed in directives from the US Conference of Catholic Bishops, to newborn resuscitation. The religion—or lack thereof—of the patient or the provider does not matter; at a Catholic hospital, everyone is treated as if they were Catholic. The directives "prohibit a range of reproductive health services, including contraception, sterilization, many infertility treatments, and abortion care, even when a woman's health or life is in danger. They can interfere with the care a woman receives if she is miscarrying and prohibit intervention even into ectopic pregnancies. Moreover, the Directives often restrict even the ability of hospital staff to provide patients with full information and referrals for care that conflict with [Catholic] religious teachings."[47]

The directives do not address newborn resuscitation explicitly, leaving the practice open to some interpretation. The Bishops' *Ethical and Religious Directives for Catholic Health Care Services* states the following:

> A person has a moral obligation to use ordinary or proportionate means of preserving his or her life. Proportionate means are those that in the

judgment of the patient offer a reasonable hope of benefit and do not entail an excessive burden or impose excessive expense on the family or the community.

A person may forgo extraordinary or disproportionate means of preserving life. Disproportionate means are those that in the patient's judgment do not offer a reasonable hope of benefit or entail an excessive burden or impose excessive expense on the family or the community.[48]

The devil is in the directives' details. What in modern, technically advanced, exceedingly expensive neonatal care is an "excessive burden" or an "excessive expense," such that the hospital would be required to provide it? The adult patient can choose for herself when to decline treatment, provided the choice is not to commit suicide. The calculus is different for impaired infants, who cannot speak for themselves and whose interests may be considered adverse to their parents. In these cases, a Catholic ethicist, who may be a priest or nun, will be consulted as to how to comply with the bishops' orders.

When considering a recently born but very sick infant, the directives are interpreted by Catholic ethicists as obligating Catholic hospitals to encourage families "to do what they can" to ensure the baby lives, given the hopeful potential that the infant could live for days or weeks.[49] According to an article in the *Catholic Lawyer*, those working in Catholic hospitals should resuscitate all babies, no matter how compromised and no matter how much harm may come from the resuscitation itself, so that determinations regarding their ongoing treatment can be deferred to a time and place other than the delivery room.[50] Then, NICU care "could be offered for a fixed time, such as one week, to allow the progress of the child to be more carefully assessed."[51]

The bishops' directives frightened me. It would be a living nightmare to watch my twins being forced alive in order, soon thereafter, for them to struggle and die painfully. I feared that a priest, who would never have to raise his own children, would decide that I, as a Catholic woman, must consent to care for two blind, mentally disabled children, made that way by forced, repetitive resuscitation. Therefore, I would do whatever I could to avoid giving birth at a Catholic hospital.

Whether a hospital is Catholic is not immediately evident. Having "Holy" or "Saint" in the hospital's name is a good tip-off, but it is not an infallible approach; consider, for example, Georgetown or University of Detroit, which are also Catholic. In 2016, the Catholic Church controlled one in every six acute care hospital beds in the United States; 14.5 percent of all acute care hospitals in the United States are Catholic owned or affiliated.[52] With mergers and acquisitions, the church has consolidated its ownership of competing hospitals, so what is not Catholic today may be Catholic tomorrow. Between 2001 and 2016 the number of Catholic-sponsored or -affiliated hospitals increased by 22 percent.[53]

A patient also may not have the luxury of choosing a hospital provider. Over the last decade, from 2001, while the church increased its possession of American hospitals, the overall number of hospitals nationwide declined.[54] The dead zone of hospitals is particularly acute in rural states, where, as of 2014, 54 percent of counties do not have a hospital with obstetrics services.[55] Only one hospital may be available within miles of a laboring woman's home, and that hospital may be Catholic. Or if a family calls an ambulance to transport a pregnant patient urgently needing medical care, the ambulance will take the patient to the closest hospital or one where the ambulance company has a contract. The patient, who has assiduously sought to avoid Catholic healthcare, may nevertheless find herself at a Catholic-run facility and subject to their dogma-infused policies.

The DC area has an embarrassment of medical riches as home to a dozen hospitals with labor and delivery wards. Nine hospitals have NICUs, but only Children's National Hospital has a Level 5 NICU, complete with helipad. Because it is a hospital for children, however, it does not have a labor and delivery ward and does not support births. Newborn babies are transported there (often by helicopter, which would land on the roof helipad), and parents cannot stay with their babies.

Three hospitals within easy driving distance from my home had Level 4 NICUs, but two of these hospitals are Catholic and would have, I presumed, mandatory resuscitation policies. I telephoned the administrators at each Catholic hospital to learn the specifics of their requirements for newborn resuscitation—and I got nowhere. The Catholic hospitals' management would not reveal their policies; they would not even confirm or deny the existence of a mandatory resuscitation rule. They kept repeating that newborn care decisions would be made as a team with the hospital staff, my doctors, and me. But they would not tell me which mandatorily Catholic criteria would be applied to this decision-making.

Time to think like a lawyer. I placed calls to the other NICUs in the region, those too far away from my house to be used, although I did not reveal that fact. Instead, I told the NICU head nurses (or whomever I spoke to) that I was trying to determine where to give birth and anticipated a long NICU stay for my twins. Would they please tell me why I should choose their hospital and NICU over their competitors? Tongues were loosened immediately by providing a profit motive and an opportunity to gossip about the competition. A complicated labor and delivery plus a double NICU stay would be worth millions! All I had to do was sit back and let others tell me about the terrible policies elsewhere—but not at their august institution. NICU nurses also often move among hospitals, and if they had an axe to grind against a former employer, they were sure to let me know.

I got an earful. Nurse after nurse told me that she personally would not give birth at the Catholic hospitals in town. Even if the parents are opposed, the Catholics made at least two attempts to resuscitate every newborn. In the nurses' estimation, the Catholic insistence at resuscitation was cruel, harmful, and out of step with best practice. The secular hospitals made one attempt to resuscitate a newborn who was not breathing, or, if the parents objected, no attempt at all. My suspicions confirmed, I removed the two Catholic hospitals from consideration.

That left George Washington University Hospital. What kismet: my obstetrician had credentials to attend births at GWU. From her, I was able to ferret out the telephone number for the charge nurse in the labor and delivery ward. The nurse gave me the number to the NICU, which connected me with the head nurse there. That nurse returned my voicemail inquiring about the hospital's resuscitation policies. She was shocked that I had called; in her years of attending premature babies, no parent had ever asked about resuscitation before birthing a baby in respiratory distress. The hospital was not religious, she informed me, and further, was located in Washington, DC. No mandatory resuscitation law or doctrine applied to the hospital, so it got to make its own. GWU's own neonatal resuscitation policy was that advanced resuscitation measures would be offered to critically ill newborns only in consultation with the parents and with their consent. Eureka, I'd found it! A hospital that met my criteria for caring for me and my fragile twins. GWU had won the labor and delivery ward and NICU beauty contest. My plan was set, and I would give birth there.

When time came for the twins' birth, I would be on my own to demand a birth with as little medical intervention as possible and to battle hospital policies on forced resuscitation, this while I labored to deliver two babies. The accoutrements of birth—blood, needles, tubes, and screaming—make my spouse queasy, so he would not be present for the event. He would be camped out in the waiting room like a 1950s husband, ready to hand out cigars and whiskey shots as soon as the doctor announced, "It's a boy!" My spouse had run away from my first birth. He popped his head into the room just as the baby was crowning, was overcome with disgust, and proclaimed, "I can't do this." He then left, leaving the midwives to chase him down the hall and me alone to push out a half a baby. His personality is gruff and not comforting, as he is easily irritated by processes, such as labor and delivery, that are lengthy, messy, or do not follow a set plan. And we both would perish of mortification if he saw me splayed out, legs akimbo, with bodily fluids dripping from my genitals.

Instead, with everything else going wrong with my pregnancy, I put my faith in a complete stranger and hired a doula to keep me company during labor and safe through the birth process. A doula is an unlicensed, non-medical birth attendant who provides emotional, almost magical support to a birthing parent. Communication with and encouragement from a doula makes for better pregnancy outcomes. Mothers accompanied by a doula have significantly shorter labors and lower rates of caesarean deliveries.[56] With the doula's experienced eyes scrutinizing the birth, mothers are two times less likely to experience a birth complication involving themselves or their baby.[57] Their babies are four times less likely to be low birth weight, and they have higher Apgar scores after delivery.[58] Doula-assisted mothers are much more likely to initiate breastfeeding.[59]

Although sites such as "DONA International"[60] tout doulas' ability to guide families though childbirth, I did not seek a guide. The doula I wanted would be part advocate, part warrior, and wholly able to give a long and powerful back massage. This was a pro tip I picked up from my birthing center delivery: in the absence of pain medicine, a lower back massage will cut the mind-searing labor pain long enough for you to catch your breath, stop screaming, and not die. The first go-round, I had asked my spouse to massage my back to dull the agony. This he did for a few minutes and then got bored. Fortunately, one of the midwife-trainees attending me was also a doula. Wielding a sock filled with heated rice, she jumped into the breach to warm and knead my back muscles for hours until the baby was born. She also was not grossed out by the birth's nudity and gore, treating them both as unremarkable.

That the doula would be warm and caring company at a fraught time mattered less to me than that she would fight for me when I could no longer do so. Childbirth is such a dangerous process that there is no guarantee that women will get through it alive. In the sixteenth century queens and noblewomen would write wills in case they did not survive childbirth.[61] Though I'm no European queen, I did the same and added a living will and DNR (do not resuscitate) order for myself. Maternal mortality ratios have declined precipitously since the introduction after World War II of antibiotics and other medicines to control infections, high blood pressure, and bleeding.[62] But death or incapacitation caused by childbirth is still not uncommon, especially in the United States, which has the highest level of maternal mortality in the developed world.[63]

Childbirth can go sideways in an instant, which is why "women work with their doctors or doulas to design a birth plan describing how they want their delivery to go, what measures they are not comfortable with, and who should make decisions if they cannot."[64] I would look to my doula to help me fend off epidurals and C-sections if I became weak willed during labor. If I lost consciousness, my doula would speak for me to reject any extraordinary measures to maintain my life or that of the twins. In those critical moments, whatever plan I had penned on paper would not matter.

Hospitals in most states have no legal obligation to honor a pregnant woman's living will or DNR, although a nonpregnant person's wishes might be respected.[65] Twelve states demand that a woman be kept alive by any means necessary until her baby can be delivered safely. "In Alabama, Idaho, Indiana, Kansas, Michigan, Missouri, Oklahoma, South Carolina, Texas, Utah, Washington, and Wisconsin, a brain dead pregnant woman's vital organs can be kept functioning as long as necessary to incubate a fetus until it is developed enough for delivery—even if that is not what she or her family wanted."[66] Most of these same states (with the exception of Oklahoma and Washington, but adding Kentucky) ignore a woman's written desires not to receive artificial nutrition and hydration or mechanical ventilatory assistance for herself because the woman is pregnant.[67]

I would be giving birth in Maryland, one of only eight states that permit pregnant women to create a binding living will.[68] Just in case something should go very badly, and with my spouse absent from the delivery room, I would need someone to be my voice. I wanted to make it abundantly clear that my life took priority over my fetuses' and, if all else failed, that I should not be kept alive in a vegetative state. For this delicate and intimate hire, I of course turned to the neighborhood listserv for recommendations. Having a doula is common in my corner of the world, which is replete with homebirths and midwives. From the referrals I received, I interviewed several doulas and selected one who had a flexible schedule, so that she could respond if I went into early labor, and who had experience advocating for vaginal twin births. We met in person over cups of herbal tea to sign contracts and waivers and so I could hand over a $1,000 check. She was a calm, almost radiant woman who wore long skirts and wrist bangles and smelled slightly of patchouli.

In addition to her supportive presence during labor and delivery, the doula could provide, for a small extra fee, add-on services. She offered to collect, dry, pulverize, and encapsulate my placenta so that I could consume it afterward. Yes, mammals throughout the animal kingdom eat their placentas after giving birth, but despite recent American interest, no contemporary human culture has included traditions of eating the placenta during the postpartum period.[69] Furthermore, CDC warned against this practice after a newborn became strep infected following the mother's ingestion of her dehydrated placenta.[70] I declined these generous additional amenities. My magical thinking has its limits, and my pregnancy alone was sufficiently nausea-inducing.

Chapter Nine

Split Apart

One of the most difficult decisions in perinatal medicine is when to induce delivery of twins with sIUGR.[1] Delivering these babies too early will lead to complications associated with prematurity, including cerebral injury at birth and neonatal death, while delivering the twins too late is associated with an increased risk of single fetal death and neurological injury of the survivor or stillbirth of both fetuses.[2] At thirty-four weeks, it was time. According to my ultrasounds, the donor twin had stopped growing and was shrinking. He was, as my doctor had predicted, deteriorating. My high-risk maternal-fetal medicine specialist told me to get to the hospital within the next few days—I could wait two days but not a whole week. I would be induced, the babies would be born, and they would be rushed to the NICU.

After being known throughout the pregnancy as donor and recipient, or growth restricted and not, or little and big, my twins received new identifiers based on the order in which they would be born: Twin A and Twin B. The larger, recipient twin was Twin A, so named because he would be the first one out of me. He was standing on his head on top of my cervix, able to pop out whenever he was ready—or when the doctor decided to evict him. The smaller, donor twin was Twin B. He was in a breech position, bottom down toward my cervix, and he would be born second. The larger twin was closer to the exit, so he would push away his brother as he made grand entry to the world. Then, if all went to plan, the smaller twin would drop into the ample space created by the escaping Twin A, and out Twin B would come too.

But when had this pregnancy gone according to plan? I begged for an unmedicated, vaginal birth, which I judged the safest for me and the best and quickest route out for the babies. Although the little twin was breech, he nevertheless could, in theory, be birthed vaginally if the obstetrician were willing and able to manage the birth. But most obstetricians are opposed to supporting a vaginal twin birth—and a vaginal twin breech birth is a nonstarter. Three-quarters of twins are delivered by caesarean section in the United States, and virtually all, 92 percent, of breech twin births are C-sections.[3]

Because of the absence of clinical trials and conflicting recommendations in the medical literature, there is fierce disagreement about how twins should be birthed. Review of the latest and best data on twin deliveries, even when twins are positioned in opposite directions, like a yin and a yang, and when the twins are of discordant weights, indicates that a vaginal delivery may be the preferred exit route.[4] If any harm comes to the second twin through a vaginal delivery, it is associated with a long delay, more than half an hour, between births or with prematurity of the twins.[5]

For my own well-being, I did not want the major abdominal surgery, lengthy recovery, and adverse effects on subsequent pregnancies that a C-section would entail. I felt selfish trying to limit my own harm from delivering the twins; fortunately, the way to ensure my health and theirs was not opposed. Twins born vaginally do as well or better than those born by C-section, and poor consequences for twins born vaginally are rare. For the babies themselves, a planned vaginal delivery results in birth outcomes similar to a planned C-section.[6] This felicitous conclusion holds even when the first twin is born vaginally and the second twin must be delivered by an emergency C-section, a painful, unanticipated end for one out of every five mothers who planned vaginal births of their twins.[7]

Comparison of a large sample of vaginal and caesarean twin deliveries found no significant differences in the death rates for the babies at birth, the babies' Apgar scores, the number of babies' deaths within a month of birth, or their sickness because of lack of oxygen (asphyxia). But premature twins delivered by planned C-section suffered more, not less, prematurity-related sickness and more sickness and death related to other factors. Preemie twins of less than thirty-six weeks and six days born by a planned C-section delivery died more often immediately before or after birth, although asphyxia-related morbidity did not differ from planned vaginal births. A planned caesarean delivery was related to more sickness and death and lower Apgar scores.[8] For twins born at term, whether the babies were birthed vaginally or by C-section neither increased nor decreased the babies' sickness or death. The only benefit of a C-section was seen when a caesarean delivery was planned for twin babies over thirty-seven weeks. Planning the C-section may ensure a less chaotic emergency delivery, resulting in less asphyxia- and trauma-related outcomes for the twins.[9]

A caesarean delivery is presumptively indicated only when the "presenting," or first to be born, twin is positioned nonvertex (not head down) and cannot be enticed to turn around. My first child was positioned nonvertex at forty weeks, which was still two weeks before I delivered him. With time ticking down on the clock and determined to avoid a hospitalized birth that a breech delivery would require, I consulted an acupuncturist who claimed great success in getting babies to turn. After he stuck needles in my back, he lit a giant blunt of various herbs and waved them around my belly. That baby turned two days later, and I had a nonhospitalized birth at a birthing center. (No, there is absolutely no scientific reason why flaming plants located in the general vicinity of a uterus would cause a fetus to reposition itself. All pregnant women are susceptible to magical thinking.) With my twins, and to my everlasting regret, I was given too little notice of their birth for me to schedule an appointment with my acupuncturist.

For all twin deliveries, an obstetrician skilled in vaginal breech delivery should be present because the second twin may flip from a vertex to a breech position. The obstetrician should also know how to turn the second twin while still in the uterus by turning the baby from butt-first to headfirst or turning the baby so that its feet present first. But in only 20 percent of cases is a C-section necessary for a twin birth.[10]

So why are so many twins birthed by C-section in the United States? The almost universal prematurity of twins is used as an excuse for the blanket requirement of C-sections for twins. My medical team argued that contractions during labor would be too dangerous for premature babies, and a midwife friend added some nuance to this assertion. She explained that it is standard of care to deliver severely preterm babies by a caesarean section because of concern about trauma to the babies from being squeezed by the mother's muscles. Premature babies were adjudged to be at increased risk of internal bleeding, particularly in the brain, as their fragile capillaries can break easily. Further, preemies have minimal or no fat, believed necessary to protect their bodies from the contractions of labor.

The science does not bear out the danger to preemies of a natural birth. A review of singleton births found that a vaginal birth would be safe for babies older than twenty-four weeks.[11] For twins, even those born prematurely, birth trauma–associated morbidity for the babies was incredibly low (at 0.2 percent) after a vaginal delivery.[12] Trauma to the mothers was, of course, not measured.

Also knocked down was the argument that a C-section was necessitated by my twins' different sizes, whether caused by TTTS or sIUGR. No data supported requiring a caesarean for discordant sizes or birthweights of the twins alone. A retrospective study found twin fetus size discordance does not represent a contraindication to a vaginal "trial of labor," my most favorite phrase in all of medicine. Discordant twins do not have a higher risk of heart rate decelerations with contractions.[13] This holds true no matter which baby, the larger or the smaller, is the first to be born. Even cases of extreme discordance such as the one I was facing, in which one twin is more than 40 percent larger than the other, do not rule out labor and vaginal delivery or suggest that a C-section would ensure better birth outcomes.[14]

I argued to my doctors that I should be permitted to try to avoid a C-section, provided that each twin was considered gestationally older than the minimum gestation age for a singleton vaginal birth. My line and verse were the following: "There is an abundance of . . . observational data with several hundreds of subjects that unanimously supports the safety of vaginal delivery of the nonvertex second twin by demonstrating improved or equal neonatal outcomes compared with caesarean delivery."[15] Being unable to provide me any other scientific study or review that showed contrary evidence, my doctors agreed to let me plan for a vaginal birth. That battle won, I then turned to fighting another against medically inducing my labor and giving me an epidural of pain medications. Out again came my medical journals and summaries of studies on birth outcomes. By now, my doctors could only roll their eyes at my insistence.

The big fetus was comfortably growing inside of me, but the little fetus had to come out far ahead of either my or his schedule. If I wanted a vaginal birth, I did not have the luxury of waiting weeks for my body to spontaneously begin laboring on its own. Hormonally and physically, I wasn't ready to give birth, but a cocktail of medicines would at least put me through the motions needed to excise the babies. My uterine contractions would be induced using an intravenous drug called Pitocin (oxytocin). My still closed cervix would be softened and thinned, "ripened" like a peach, with prostaglandin suppositories shoved up my vagina.[16] Though necessary, inducing labor felt like a failure to me. In the United States, but not elsewhere, inductions of twins inevitably result in C-sections, the very outcome I sought to avoid.

The straight progression from induced labor to C-section should not occur. In singleton births, the odds are very good that a C-section can be avoided: three-quarters of inductions end in vaginal deliveries and a quarter in C-sections.[17] In fact, new information indicates inductions can reduce C-sections in singleton babies who are at term for their gestation.[18] Having twins changes these odds. Induction of twin pregnancies is associated with a twofold increase in risk of caesarean section compared with those twin pregnancies permitted to wait for the onset of spontaneous labor.[19] Still, Sweden manages to ensure that 80 percent of induced twin labors are delivered vaginally.[20] In the United States, it is quite the opposite. Induction of labor for the 25 percent of twins intended to have a vaginal birth ends with almost 40 percent delivered by C-section and all the attendant risks to the mother of blood loss and hysterectomy.[21]

The difference in the mode of twin deliveries in Sweden and the United States may be explained by the pain medications routinely used for laboring American women. Pitocin for inductions causes painful, strong contractions that come faster and faster with shorter intervals for rest or recovery. Relief is administered through an epidural, which numbs the mother from the waist down. With an epidural, the mother must labor on her back in bed, attached to a back catheter through which the pain medication is delivered. Epidurals slow the contractions, making more difficult the act of pushing out the babies, and extend the labor, making it harder to manage.[22] The combination of the epidural medications and longer labor puts more stress on the birthing infants, potentially causing their heart rate to decrease.[23] When that happens, an emergency C-section may be required to give the babies an end to the hours of squeezing and a quick exit.[24]

If I was to lose the skirmish on induction, I would win the one on unmedicated childbirth. Having already had a pain relief–free delivery with my first child, I knew I could grit my teeth and bear laboring with the twins, as unpleasant as it would be. My planned vaginal birth also included plans to wave away any anesthesiologists who offered me an epidural.

Unfortunately, the urgency of the impending birth meant neither my regular obstetrician nor the hospital she practiced at, GWU, was available. GWU's maternity ward was filled with laboring women who were giving birth at term and according to plan. In addition, my own OB was also pregnant and due at this very moment. Had I reached my due date, my doctor could have birthed her own baby, taken six weeks of maternity leave, and delivered me. This was now not possible. Nor could I simply go to any hospital or have any doctor deliver me, because the facility or the physician might not have the skill to manage my complex case or the NICU to care for the twins—or they might force me into a C-section that I had successfully advocated that I avoid. Despairing, I spent a day calling hospitals, trying to find one that could accommodate me.

My high-risk maternal-fetal specialist took pity. He found a bed for me at the Catholic hospital where his office was located. Yes, the hospital had a mandatory resuscitation policy, but he assured me that the twins were developed enough not to be harmed by it. Although he didn't usually deliver babies, being fully occupied with the care of women with complex pregnancies, he canceled his vacation with his son so he could attend to me. Many years earlier, at the beginning of his career, he had served as the medical director for Planned Parenthood of the Rocky Mountains. He had performed abortions for every woman in need in conservative states such as Utah, where no other provider was available. With Shiva-like powers, what he could destroy, he could create; what he could terminate, he could save. Initially, I was embarrassed by the thought of a male doctor viewing me naked and laboring. I quickly came around to the realization that I would be in excellent hands— and that my back was against a wall with no further choices.

My sister had come up from South Carolina to watch my toddler for the duration. We gave her a menu for the next few meals and told her to call us if she needed anything. Notwithstanding all the information and counseling the doctors had given us, we all presumed that whatever we were facing would be over in a day or so. We were like those who refuse to evacuate, hoping the hurricane bearing straight down on them will curve in its track and pass them by. By failing to plan and refusing to face reality, we attempted to will the situation to be normal and unremarkable.

The evening before I gave birth, my spouse took a picture of me in our new driveway so we could remember how not-large I was. The summer twilight lit me to my best advantage, but that these twins were not fully cooked was obvious. I looked conventionally pregnant, not about to birth two babies in less than twenty-four hours. The fetuses were small even considering that they would be more than a month premature. Yet we had no choice but to expel them. Following the photo shoot, I returned to my home office to pull an all-nighter, frantically closing and transferring work projects until I could resume them.

At some ungodly, o'dark-hundred hour in the morning, my spouse and I headed for the hospital. The house was quiet, with my sister and toddler sound asleep. As we pulled away from the house, I watched the headlights bisect the entire house and contemplated that I still hadn't even managed to hang curtains in the windows. The flash illuminated in the otherwise empty living room two baby hammocks and two automatic rocking cradles, empty and waiting.

The hospital was as empty and silent as my living room, if better lit. The parking lot was eerily empty, without its usual crush of taxis with passengers still stoned postsurgery. Although it was the largest hospital in the region with supposedly the busiest maternity ward, we were the only couple in the waiting room.

I surreptitiously breakfasted on granola bars, apples, and water, confident that I would not need a caesarean section, so the hospital's asinine restrictions on eating did not apply to me. The presumption at hospitals is that a childbirth will end with a C-section, so presurgical fasting protocols must be followed. The fear is that the mother, if she has any food in her stomach, will inhale her vomit when put under anesthesia. No thought is given to the caloric needs to sustain the intense, aerobic exercise of birth over multiple hours or that birth is a long, slow process, taking place during the span of time most people would eat two or three meals. Again, hospitals seek to limit their perceived liability, although there is little evidence to support policies that prohibit laboring mothers from eating. In fact, the data show that there is no harm to women from eating and drinking while in labor, that women voluntarily choose to stop eating and drinking as labor progresses, and that maternal comfort is improved by allowing consumption of food and water during the childbirth process.[25] Also overstated are concerns about women aspirating their vomit: a review of 720,000 births requiring the use of anesthesia found one case of vomit aspiration.[26]

After I'd munched my way through my feed bag, my doula showed up—late, I noted, but late for what? An hour after arriving, we still were sitting, waiting. My spouse groused that he was hungry and wanted to find the cafeteria. Finally, my doctor materialized, finishing a yogurt, and a nurse called me back to the labor suite. They seemed surprised when I waved off my husband and told him that I would see him in a few hours. "He doesn't do childbirth," I explained and introduced everyone to my doula. The doctor exchanged phone numbers with my spouse so he could text him updates on my condition.

My previous birthing center birth had not prepared me for the awkwardness of a complicated hospital-based birth. As a preliminary matter, I was instructed to disrobe and put on a hospital gown that covered absolutely nothing—not my breasts, not my rear, not my protruding belly, not my unkempt pubis, which I had never gotten around to waxing during my truncated birth preparations. Witnessing my striptease were a crowd of strangers: my doula, three or four nurses, and three doctors. Soon, a medical school class joined them. These ten or so students had been promised a show involving an unmedicated, vaginal birth of twins, one of whom would require a breech extraction. The cost of admission was witnessing a disheveled, naked woman scream obscenities for several hours. No one inquired whether I consented to this many people seeing my most private body parts, but by then it was as if I had disappeared. Everyone was there to see the twins; their current home was of no interest.

Much like my pregnancy, the birth did not go according to plan. The spectacle was hardly the heartwarming miracle of life the medical students had lined up to see. My labor was medically induced. For hours, nothing happened except the odd, painful contraction, which caused me to curse theatrically. More and more Pitocin was given, and my contractions piled onto one another, with no relief in between. I could only howl in pain, and my doula's attempts at backrubs or warm compresses were wholly ineffectual. The doula suggested that a hot shower might dull the stabbing in my back and crotch, but I could not stand up straight in the water. My hospital gown was soaked, my hair disheveled, my legs covered in blood and mucus. I crawled between the bed and bathroom, snarling and shrieking like a trapped banshee.

Finally, one of the nurses had enough. She demanded that I put into laboring the energy I was wasting screaming. I do not know how I would have managed to give birth in a different country or a culture that demands that the laboring mother does not wail from the pain. In the former Soviet Union, where I had spent three years working in maternal healthcare, mothers are expected to labor and birth silently.[27] Nurses will slap violators across their faces to enforce a hospital edict of no sound at delivery. A screaming woman is presumed to be a bad mother who is traumatizing her baby.

Larger Twin A was born vaginally after twelve hours of unmedicated labor, when the nurses and doctors finally wrestled me into the hospital bed for the delivery. He was in respiratory distress as he emerged and made no sound. He was shown to me long enough for me to verify that he was living and to see that, as the TTTS recipient, he was very dark colored. A doctor asked me to name Twin A, but I couldn't remember any of the names I had selected. Because my husband wasn't present for the birth, I couldn't ask him what name we had agreed on. Through a fog of pain, I grasped for a familiar name— Francis! That must be it. A pediatrician bundled up Frankie and ran with him out the door. Only later did I realize that I had inadvertently named my child for the Pope. In my lowest moments, you could take the girl out of the Church, but not the Catholic Church out of the girl.

Certainly, Twin B would be on his way out any second. The doula, the OBs, the group of medical students, the nurses, and I used the interstitial time to decide Twin B's name. By now, my contractions had slowed, and I could think more clearly. The options were Frederick, a family name from an ancient relative who was Napoleon's cannoneer, or Declan, which, I now recalled, was what I had called Frankie in utero. The choices were put to a vote of those assembled. The nurses asked the head OB to vote first—and all eyes were on him as he declared that Frederick was too harsh sounding for a little baby (and more appropriate for an Alsatian soldier). He cast a lot for Declan, and the rest of the room respected the hospital hierarchy. By a unanimous vote, Twin B was to be named Declan.

Declan did not want to be born. I pushed and pushed until I felt my intestines reverse themselves and hemorrhoids pop out. To my horror, I pooped on the delivery table. My humiliation was complete. Many years earlier, I had found on my best friend's shelf ex–Playboy Playmate Jenny McCarthy's book about birth.[28] McCarthy dedicated a full chapter to describing her fears of defecating during childbirth and her attempts to avoid it. She too had heard of the possibility of pushing until you poop, so she was careful to use an enema to clean herself out before being induced. Playboy Bunnies are comely with their clothes on or off, and McCarthy ensured the view remained pleasant for those who had to witness her giving birth.

Other sources far more reliable than that of a vaccine denier suggest that "most" people in labor are unable to control their rectums.[29] Women are reassured that defecating while pushing is wholly natural and even desirable, indicating that the proper muscles are engaged in pushing and that nothing would block the baby's emergence from the birth canal. For me, it was merely revolting. I had no access to an enema in the mad run-up to what was becoming a catastrophic childbirth. Too late I realized I shouldn't have eaten those granola bars or that apple, which, over the intervening twelve hours, had traversed my alimentary tract and emerged from the other end. One of the labor and delivery nurses swooped in to scoop up the mess. Everyone was polite enough not to mention it, and I tried not to make eye contact with my doctors.

Still no Declan. He had swum upward inside of me and was stuck somewhere under my ribs. The doctor found him at the top of my uterus on his portable ultrasound machine. No amount of pushing would dislodge him, and I had pushed until I had no strength left. My own doctor sharply ordered the room cleared of all nonessential personnel, and medical students quickly scuttled out like a fluffle of frightened rabbits. A spinal block was ordered, and as it took effect, a revelation: I was no longer in horrendous pain. I wondered to a nurse whether most people used medicine to reduce the pain of their contractions. The nurse regarded me as if I were an alien from Mars and said, curtly, "Yes." Oh. So that's how they do it.

Two doctors donned shoulder-length gloves and plexiglass eye shields and dove into me to look for Twin B. Each had an arm inside of me, fishing around. Once, my doctor caught the baby's arm and tried to squeeze out the rest of him. No luck, and away he swam. I began to bleed and looked through my legs to find my doctors covered in red splatter. The head doctor shouted to move me—fast—into surgery. A team of people in scrubs rushed me down the hall to the operating theater, a river of blood flowing behind us.

Each year around the world, more than a third of a million women die from pregnancy and childbirth. These mothers' lives end because they have created new life and have been rewarded with infections, high blood pressure, and hemorrhage for their trouble. Of these causes, hemorrhage, uncontrolled bleeding, is the leading cause of maternal death globally.[30] The condition is responsible for between 25 and 60 percent of birth-related deaths.[31] The woman's life flows away in a red gush of never-ending blood, often in the final stage of labor or immediately after the baby is born.

Malawi, the project site for my maternal and child health nonprofit, has some of the highest death rates from postpartum hemorrhage. Approximately one woman dies for every hundred babies born alive, and a quarter of these maternal deaths are from excessive bleeding.[32] If birth attendants knew how to stop a woman's bleeding, or if there was blood to give her to replace what she had lost, the woman would live. But in Malawi, there are no doctors to attend births. There are few nurses. And there certainly isn't blood to transfuse a woman who has bled out because there's not even electricity to keep stored blood refrigerated. Women labor alone; when they start to bleed, they die alone.

Compared with Malawi, few American women die hemorrhaging in childbirth. But our country's statistics on maternal mortality are deplorable—and downright frightening if you happen to be a health policy expert who is, at that very moment, bleeding excessively while trying to give birth. More disconcerting is if you are laboring, gushing blood, and located in the District of Columbia, whose maternal death rates are almost twice the US national average and are on par with those in a developing country.[33] Giving birth is one of the most dangerous, life-threatening activities a Black woman in DC could undertake. For every hundred thousand births in the US capital, sixty Black women die from pregnancy or childbirth, at the same ratio of live babies to dead moms as in Kyrgyzstan,[34] another country not known for laudable maternal healthcare and where I had lived.

Again, I was fortunate: I was not located in Malawi or Kyrgyzstan or even DC. My hospital was one mile north of the District border. In Maryland, women are much more likely to have their hemorrhages managed effectively and thus to survive childbirth. Furthermore, I am white, not Black, and although naked, I was cloaked in an invisible shield of privilege. I would receive competent and solicitous hospital care and my childbirth story would ultimately be a happy one.

My hired doula held my hand as I dry heaved—but did not aspirate vomit!—from the anesthesia for an emergency C-section. I was freezing cold, exhausted, depressed, and wanted to go home. Leaving became a single-minded obsession. I decided that I was finished with childbirth for the day and that I would walk home. But I was trapped, strapped to a gurney for surgery. My legs no longer responded because of my spinal block. Yet every cell in me screamed, "Run away! Run away!" Tears streamed down my face as I was filleted like a fish. I smelled my skin as it was cut and felt my intestines and organs pulled and tugged. Birth was not beautiful; it was awful, and it was lonely.

Two-and-a-half hours after Twin A's birth and just before midnight, Twin B finally was lifted out of me. He weighed less than three pounds, but he managed a small cry, almost like a kitten's mew. "A little peanut!" exclaimed one of the pediatricians who showed me a tiny body wrapped in a receiving blanket. I briefly glimpsed Declan before he was whisked away to the NICU. Frankie, Twin A and TTTS recipient, had been black with blood. Declan, Twin B and the TTTS donor, was pale white.

There was nothing more to do than to put my intestines back where they belonged and to sew me up. The doctors finished their work and bid me goodnight. I said an awkward goodbye to my doula, with whom I've not communicated since and whom I almost certainly underpaid for all her trouble. What is the appropriate hourly rate for almost eighteen hours of observing, hearing, and smelling viscera and gore? An orderly wheeled me upstairs to my empty, overpriced hospital hotel room. I was spent and wanted to curl up and sleep for several days to forget the whole ordeal. Instead, per bizarre hospital policy, I was awakened every two hours for unnecessary checks of my blood sugar. At daybreak, I inquired whether I could see the babies; I could not. They were not in a state to be viewed. Several floors above the babies who no longer resided in me, I lay in a rented bed and stared at the ceiling.

Twelve hours after I gave birth, a nurse rolled me in a wheelchair to the NICU. Frankie and Declan looked like laboratory specimens stored in separate test tubes. Cords and lines ran in all directions from their tiny bodies: breathing tubes, feeding tubes, IVs, heart monitors, and thermometers. Frankie's lungs were inflated by a ventilator. Declan lay on a special air mattress to protect his delicate skin. Both wore the tiniest, origami-folded, preemie diapers ever seen outside a dollhouse. Only days later was I permitted to hold them.

NICUs sound like casinos and are as filled with desperation. Alarms sound every few seconds, but instead of heralding a jackpot, these usually mean a baby's lungs have stopped breathing or heart has ceased beating. Babies are displayed in transparent containers and intubated every which way. If they cry or scream from pain or loneliness, the babies can hardly be heard. The closed-in incubators muffle the sound, and the alarms obscure it. Parents, many of whom resemble the sleepless, walking dead, stand watch at the foot of their babies' incubators or kangaroo their babies to their bare chests, trying simultaneously to maintain the babies' body temperatures without loosening a tube or cord—resulting in another alarm. I asked a NICU nurse how she could stand to work in such a stressed, distressing atmosphere. She responded that NICUs' successes are so many more than their failures. To her, NICUs are happy places where babies are grown and medical personnel perform daily miracles.

The "glass is half full" view of NICUs is the more positive way of thinking about the frightening, exhausting ordeal that is inherent in having newborn children in a NICU. The facts, however, are that a fragile infant who has survived childbirth still must survive a stay in neonatal intensive care, and the challenges to survival are many. The conditions that end or damage tiny lives just begun are standard in all NICUs: necrotizing enterocolitis, retinopathy of prematurity, infections, and brain bleeds. But while NICU patients' trials are well studied, different NICUs have vastly different sickness and death outcomes.[35] Something inherent to the treatment received at one NICU versus another determines whether a baby eventually goes home healthy—or ever leaves the hospital alive. By now, having learned lessons from genetic testing through CVS, TTTS treatment, fetoscopic laser surgery, and high-risk labor and delivery, I could anticipate part of the answer to what translates into NICU survival: specialization and volume. Higher-level NICUs have fewer neonatal deaths than lower-level NICUs, and NICUs that serve many patients have better outcomes than those that have fewer than fifty admissions per year.[36]

NICUs' competition for patients is fierce, as charges for a single baby's multiweek stay in the facility can exceed a million dollars. Yet using advertising and promotional inducements to push maternity patients to hospitals with lower level NICUs comes at the expense of the survival and well-being of babies. Studies conducted since the 1990s have consistently demonstrated that "mortality rates are higher among preterm infants born in hospitals with a low-level or midlevel NICU than among those born in hospitals with a high-level NICU."[37] More recent information indicates that, although doctors and equipment can be disbursed to smaller local hospitals, these human and mechanical resources cannot overcome a dearth of experience in saving babies' lives. Among the infants born in hospitals with less than fifty deliveries per year, the odds of death or severe brain hemorrhage in particular were 15 to 36 percent higher after adjusting for NICU level.[38] Fortunately, the NICU where Frankie and Declan were resident was the largest and most active in the state, and it was highly specialized, a Level IV.

Beyond having the experience and ability to treat vulnerable newborns, NICUs need to control for a common set of process problems that drive poor health outcomes.[39] In the NICUs with the highest rates of sickness and death, human breast milk feeding is too low and artificial formula use too high, medication too frequent, days spent on ventilators too many, babies' temperatures on admission too low, and attention to infection prevention too scant. The very interventions that are considered the standard of NICU care to save babies' lives immediately after birth come with considerable complications in the medium and longer term.[40] Intravenous feeding and artificial formula feeding can lead to necrotizing enterocolitis, a fatal condition if not cured promptly and surgically. Kidney and liver injury can result from use of nonsteroidal anti-inflammatory drugs (NSAIDs), antibiotics, and intravenous nutrition. Mechanical ventilation can increase the risk for intraventricular hemorrhage (brain bleeds), associated with poor neurodevelopmental outcomes. Supplemental oxygen administration can lead to retinopathy of prematurity, a common cause of blindness in premature infants. Extended stays in the NICU with central lines and IVs put infants with already vulnerable immune systems at risk for sepsis. Better neonatal care depends on tackling these problems together and as a group, rather than picking only one issue of focus at a time.

Beyond experience and specialization, the other component of NICU survival is, surprisingly, taken from change management, a dry discipline about guiding people and organizations through difficult changes in which I got certified to improve my job prospects. I would never have thought to consult it for maternal and infant health answers, but it was if the entirety of my background could be brought to bear on the conundrum of my TTTS twins. At hospitals committed to improving neonatal outcomes, the percentage of babies who died in the NICU decreased between 2007 and 2013 from over 10 percent to around 8 percent.[41] Survival through the first twenty-four hours is determinative. Except for the most premature babies (born at 23 weeks or less), if a baby lives through the first day after birth, the odds are that the baby will make it out of the NICU alive, especially at a high-volume, high-level NICU.[42]

Perceptions united with science would give my twins, or any NICU baby, the best chance of survival. Creating a sense of urgency is the most important step to transforming NICU outcomes.[43] Where doctors and nurses could see and compare their outcomes against other NICUs, and where quality failures were highlighted, policy change supportive of process improvements followed. Call it "name and shame" or "healthy competition," no NICU, hospital, or clinical team wanted the reputation of using less than the best evidence-based practices to save infants' lives. My contribution to this effort would be to continue to point out what the latest research showed and where its application was falling short.

My sister and our nanny brought my toddler to visit me in the hospital. I had never been away from him for a night, and he was understandably confused about why I had disappeared one evening and not returned home for days. He also was completely uninterested in seeing any new babies, but riding up and down the hallway in my wheelchair had its charms. While he and I were popping wheelies in the maternity ward, the other visitors snuck off to the NICU to see the twins. They returned in shock, trying to stifle their tears. Our nanny had a NICU baby years earlier, and viewing mine in their incubators and with their tubes induced posttraumatic stress. My sister was pregnant with her first and had confronted her nightmares in the flesh.

In addition to her red nose and eyes, I noticed my sister had an ugly, red welt on her wrist. A burn, she said, from trying to steam the curtains she had hung in my living room windows.

(*Chapter Ten*)

Home

Five days after birth, I was discharged from the hospital. My stay was lengthy because of my hemorrhage birthing Declan and because of complications from the C-section. I had lost so much blood that I was abjectly anemic. My doctors hesitated to transfuse me, though, for reasons I have never fully understood. I was to drink enough water to make more blood, but I must have failed in this basic duty. I remain chronically anemic to this day. My stored iron supply is nonexistent; even with years of iron supplementation and cooking my meals in an iron skillet, I've never been able to replenish it.

During his heroic efforts to save Declan, my obstetrician had inadvertently "nicked" an intestine. Ordinarily, a mother is deemed fit to leave the hospital when she poops after giving birth. With blood loss and attempts to initiate lactation, I was completely dehydrated and could not poop. With the sliced intestine, a perianal tear, a C-section slash across my abdomen, and vaginal and anal hemorrhoids, the mere concept of defecating was like sticking another knife in my already julienned undercarriage. The nurses insisted I try, and they inquired about my progress three times a day. Finally, at the end of the fifth day, a hospital billing representative informed me that my insurance would no longer cover my stay, and I was unceremoniously booted from the maternity ward. I still hadn't pooped, but the nursing staff had suddenly lost interest in this progress measure of my maternal health.

Usually, there is a celebration when a new mother departs the hospital. She is wheeled through the labor and delivery ward, her baby on her lap, the other parent proudly pushing her, balloons flying around her, flowers falling in her wake. There is no joy being discharged while your babies are in the NICU. I still could not walk, and with my spouse at home with my two-year-old, I had no one to push my wheelchair. So I hobbled doubled over and alone to the hospital exit, dragging my overnight bag and rented hospital breast pump behind me. With a crowd of visitors, I waited awkwardly for a ride, as I was prohibited from driving post-C-section. No one congratulated me on my newborns, and I left my babies behind when my father picked me up from the front of the hospital and drove me home.

Frankie and Declan stayed together in the NICU for almost three weeks. Laid out side by side in adjoining space capsule–like cribs, they did not incubate together, although they had so recently been wombmates and had shared the entirety of their fetal existence. Split apart, the twins looked so small and lonely; separating them was a most unnatural act. I inquired about cobedding, which I thought would especially benefit Declan. He had so little body fat that he lacked even a butt—his diaper covered an exit hole but no round, dimpled baby bottom—and his body temperature was dangerously low. The hospital's practice, however, was to keep each baby, even twins and triplets, in a separate bed, and I could not point to any study or data to overrule it.[1]

Both twins were treated for jaundice, dressed as tiny glowworms wrapped in cocoons embedded with blue lights. Frankie's jaundice was especially pernicious because of the blood he had filched from Declan. The extra blood cells broke down, creating bilirubin that overwhelmed his liver. Frankie's yellow skin and eyes were his entry ticket to the full tanning spa experience of days of wearing tiny sunglasses and baking naked in a heated pod of ultraviolet rays. Also jaundiced because of an immature liver, Declan additionally had an opposite problem from his twin, whose jaundice was consequent from excess. Born devoid of adequate blood, Declan had his first blood transfusions for severe anemia.

Causes célèbres in the NICU, the twins were a regular teaching exhibit on the doctors' grand rounds, with a parade of physicians marching by daily and stopping to huddle around their incubators. The babies offered something to virtually all medical subspecialties: neonatologists and pediatricians, of course, but also neurologists, audiologists, ophthalmologists, and infectious disease specialists. A geneticist stopped in and, after viewing Declan, suggested I get him, but not Frankie, tested for genetic mutations. He could not believe the twins were identical. They began their weekly appointments with a cardiologist because, as their fetal ultrasounds prognosticated, Frankie had a hole in his right ventricle and Declan's aorta was kinked.

To be sprung from the NICU clink, a baby has to demonstrate fitness to enter society. The NICU nurses say their little wards may leave A.F.T.E.R. meeting milestones on antibiotics, feeding, temperature, events, and respiration.[2] A baby must no longer require antibiotics to control infections. The baby must be able to suckle and to tolerate formula or breast milk so as to fatten up and gain the weight necessary to maintain her temperature. Relatedly, the baby must obtain temperature homeostasis, having neither an infection resulting in fever nor chills or such shivering that too many calories are expended trying to stay warm in an open crib. The baby must be on her best behavior for at least twenty-four hours, going a day without an "incident" of stopping breathing or failing to have a steady heartbeat. And the baby should be able to breathe on her own, not requiring supplemental oxygen.

The twins were given antibiotics IVs for sepsis and fed my pumped breast milk via feeding tubes through their noses. After eighteen days, Frankie was deemed able to maintain his temperature and gain weight by breastfeeding. He no longer needed a vent to breathe. He was discharged, and although I tried to negotiate keeping him a bit longer in the hospital with Declan, the nurses told me to bring Frankie home.

Having a newborn twin at home and a newborn twin in the NICU requires a mother to clone herself—or, at least, the important parts. For the next seventeen days, every three hours, I nursed Frankie out of one breast and pumped the other side. Then, leaving the bottle of pumped milk at home, I drove to the NICU, where I nursed Declan from one side and pumped the other. I'd return home and repeat. To the NICU to repeat. Back to home, back to the NICU. Day and night. In my delirium, I looked down and believed I'd grown a third breast. Instead of being disturbed, I was delighted. There it was—a pair and a spare! I had been searching all over for another breast, which certainly would ease the simultaneous nursing and pumping.

The twins' NICU was the busiest in all of Maryland, and it was a mess. The sink in front of the secured locked doors worked only half the time. When it had water at all, the water was cold and there was no soap. Visitors had to sanitize their hands the best they could before entering to see their tiny, fragile, immunocompromised infants. Inside the NICU, incubators were crowded next to cribs with inches between them. Parents took turns using the few rockers to hold their babies; nonparents stood, as no chairs were available.

Competition for the breast pumps was fierce, with the number of breasts to be expressed (a recounting determined mine were only two and not my dreamed-for three) outnumbering the available pumps. There was not enough of anything for anyone: not enough thermometers, not enough diapers or onesies, not enough privacy, too little space. From what I could tell, there was little urgency to improve or change.

The other parents feigned polite deafness when the mother six feet away was informed her child had Down syndrome. We became temporarily blind when the nurses reprimanded a teenager for forgetting, once again, to bring a car seat so she could take her baby home. When the teen left, we quietly rummaged through our babies' belongings to donate clothes and blankets to her baby who, it was already obvious, would have a life of privation. When emergency intubations or intravenous line installations had to be performed on a tiny NICU inmate, all adults were ushered to the waiting room. We shuffled silently out the door in shared terror that our own children would be the next to suffer a setback.

Declan was struggling. His heart malformation prevented him from gaining weight, even with my breast milk and formula supplementation through a feeding tube. He remained severely anemic and required another two blood transfusions. His skin color was green and mottled with infection, and a central intravenous catheter was threaded up his femoral vein at his groin to deliver antibiotics all the way to his heart. He couldn't maintain his body temperature, so he was returned to a glassed-in incubator from an open crib.

Most concerning were Declan's repeated episodes of apnea and bradycardia, where he would stop breathing and his heart rate would drop. In these instances, the monitors attached to him would shriek, and nurses and doctors would rush to resuscitate Declan. Every second mattered, as his brain and heart were starved of oxygen. But twice, when a nonresponsive, nonbreathing Declan needed air forced into him so his heart would restart, the lifesaving medical equipment was broken. The manual ventilator, located at the head of Declan's incubator, was cracked and would not inflate. The ventilator that should have been by the neighboring baby's incubator was missing in action. Hospital staff ran for an electric ventilator, but once they wheeled it over and opened it, they discovered it had a dead battery. Time ticked away, and the nurses and doctors scurried in circles in search of a new battery. As my baby turned blue, my legal training gave me the presence of mind to film the ensuing debacle of hospital staff unable to find functioning resuscitation equipment. I saved the video on my cell phone; it remains there still.

On August 17, the twins' due date, Declan was paroled from the NICU. His temperature was stable in an open crib, and his breathing and heart rate had remained steady for several days. If he could maintain his weight gain, he could be cared for at home; if he retrogressed, he would be readmitted to the NICU. He failed one criterion for freedom, however. He still weighed an ounce shy of four pounds, the minimum weight for an infant car seat. This metric was jettisoned in a push to gain Declan his freedom. The NICU nurses taught me to roll baby blankets around Declan to stabilize him in his car seat, and they wished us well.

Declan and Frankie were reunited at home. They didn't seem to notice one another at all—until that night, when both woke every two hours, screaming in unison for milk. Their stomachs were so little that they could not retain enough food to sleep for longer periods. I rolled over in bed, plucked both babies out of their cradles, and tandem nursed them. Then I rediapered them, dripped antibiotics in their mouths, put them back to bed at an incline to control their acid reflux and close enough to me so I could hear if they stopped breathing, and began the process anew the next hour. We all made it exactly one night together before my spouse put his foot down. His sleep had been disturbed by the nonstop wailing, suckling, and pooping. Without sleep, he couldn't work, and without his work, our bills would not get paid. Realizing he would not make it through months of sleepless nights and discovering that I was unwilling to shoulder alone the entire burden of nighttime duties, he insisted we retain a team of nurses to assist.

A friend who had married minor European royalty was the one who first advised that I hire a night nurse to help with the twins. Awash with pregnancy hormones, I was affronted by the very suggestion. For the second time in this pregnancy, I found myself arguing that I was not one of the queens of Europe, and I could not pawn the crown jewels to pay for someone else to care for my children. My friend graciously ignored me and went to work on my spouse. "Mortgage your house if you must," she said, to pay for the nurses. She insisted it would be the best decision we would ever make. While we slept, someone else would handle the bihourly feedings and, once the babies were big enough, the sleep training.

I remained opposed. Having hired help was not how my spouse or I was raised. Yes, I had agreed to having a nanny, but everyone I knew in DC had one. Night nurses were just too much and the babies, too young. My mother stayed home to care for her babies. I suppose a grandmother or friend or someone must have helped out when we were newborns. My husband was raised on a farm with thirty-five aunts and uncles and a hundred first cousins; there was always an extra set of hands. Now, no grandparents lived within five hundred miles of us. I couldn't ask my friends to stop working to take over a feeding shift, and they would have declined my request had I made it. A few of my friends had visited the twins in the NICU and recoiled in horror at their tiny, sickly appearance. No one else wanted to be responsible for accidentally dropping or breaking these fragile infants.

When I hefted the twins in their separate bucket car seats for their day-one, post-NICU pediatrics visit, I discovered that Declan had lost weight during his twenty-four hours away from the hospital. The pediatrician prepared to readmit Declan to the hospital. Unsupported and trying to do it all myself, it had taken me only hours to fail. I posed the question to the pediatrician: how did normal people keep up with the all-night feedings, hi-calorie formula making, antibiotics dosing, breathing and heart monitoring, and medicine administration for preemie twins? At least when one twin was in the NICU, I could get a couple of hours of sleep a night. But it had been over two days since I last slept, and I was already seeing double. The pediatrician stared at me for a long minute, scribbled something on her prescription pad, tore off the note, and handed me the most valuable document in my personal history: an order for nursing care for the twins. I had a face-saving way to hire the night nurses my spouse wanted.

Even if a doctor requires you to have them, finding nurses to provide newborn home care in Washington, DC, is almost an impossible task. The social worker from the twins' NICU assumed the task of finding a home nurse for the twins. She and I did an internet search of possibilities, divided them between us, and started calling. Nothing. Nothing. Nothing. Had we lived in Maryland, we would not have had a problem, but no one was licensed in DC to provide newborn care.

The dearth of home-based, pediatric nursing care in DC was odd, given its abundance in Maryland and Virginia.[3] One could conclude that DC's licensing requirements are too stringent and difficult to meet. DC law requires home health aides either to be registered nurses (or licensed practical nurses) or to have completed a certification examination.[4] Licensure must be renewed every two years, and home health aides must complete twenty-four hours of continuing education to remain able to practice.[5] Yet the home healthcare aide licensing standards in Maryland are more rigorous than those in DC, which applies only the most basic federal requirements.[6]

Something else, perhaps reputational bias, restricts the local pediatric nursing labor market. DC ranks as the worst place in the United States to be a nurse. The pay is lousy, and the cost of licensing renewals too high to make worthwhile the low pay for home health aides. As a result, there are more nursing jobs that go unfilled than anywhere else in the country.[7] By my last count, two nursing care companies provide DC home care for the aged and the disabled. The hassle and liability of caring for newborns is so great, though, that few nurses are willing to assume the responsibility.

Yet the scuttlebutt on the invaluable neighborhood listserv revealed a whole industry of baby night nurses from innovatively named companies like "Hush, Hush Little Baby" and "Let Mommy Sleep." These folks appear to command top dollar, anywhere from $25 to $30 an hour. What gives? Most "nurses" are not individuals who are registered nurses but are instead unlicensed care providers—doulas! That's how mothers avoid the awkward goodbyes to the person who had seen them naked and shitting as they gave birth: the labor and delivery doula becomes a postpartum doula to help with the baby at home.

Just as with their labor and delivery work, postpartum doulas exist in a grey zone of regulation. No license is required to feed, diaper, and rock a baby to sleep, and postpartum doulas confine themselves to these activities. Without a license as an actual nurse or home health aide, they may not record a baby's weight or administer medications.

Practically and financially, I could not hire a postpartum doula. My baby was going to be re-NICU'd unless I could induce him to gain weight, necessitating constant weight monitoring on a hospital-grade scale. Both twins were immunocompromised and received multiple syringefuls daily of amoxicillin and other antibiotics. To stop him from regurgitating his food and losing those calories needed for growth, Declan additionally required a titration of acid reflux medicine. The dosage had to be so finely calibrated that both his pediatrician and the pharmacist had incorrectly calculated it. Again drawing on the ever-faithful Dr. Google and my two semesters of university chemistry classes, I had found and corrected the error before I poisoned my child. But as a public health professional, I was not going to put my children's lives in the hands of a poorly trained paraprofessional. As an attorney, I wanted the law on my side in case I had to sue someone.

How I found Mary and her Baby Rockers nurses is fuzzy, as is everything from those initial days of having both babies at home. It was word of mouth, I think, thanks to the cosmopolitan melting pot that is DC. Our Salvadoran nanny knew a Togolese nanny who, through the West African diaspora, knew Mary because she was Ghanaian. Mary managed a group of African women, immigrants from Ghana, Tanzania, and Kenya, all licensed practical nurses or registered nurses in the United States who were inexplicably working as postpartum doulas. What Mary had in nursing experience and potential to break into the market for skilled infant care, she lacked in business acumen. She had never applied for a business license in DC, her license in Maryland had expired, and she was constantly losing nurses because of her accounting errors with their salaries.

I struck a deal with Mary: if she would give me a break on the cost of caring for the twins each night, I would ensure the legal compliance of her business. I renewed her business licenses and registered her as a home healthcare company in DC. I developed for her an invoice template that met insurance company standards and a business plan for her to formalize a connection with local NICUs. I coached her on presenting her business to the area hospitals so, when parents were discharged with fragile newborns, they could receive a referral to Mary and her team.

Then, for eight months, Mary or another of her nurses lived in our basement. In another strike of serendipity, the house we accidently bought in the wrong state had the perfect in-law suite to accommodate the nurses we did not know we would need. They would arrive at 10 p.m., when they would collect the babies and the accoutrements for their care, and, if the nurses woke up in time, would depart at 6 a.m. Twice, initially, and then once nightly, I would wake and pump bottles of breast milk for the nurses' use the following night. At dawn, I would tip-toe downstairs and spirit away two babies for nursing. Mary, snoring like a power saw and exhausted from her night labors, would sleep the morning away.

Financially, once nurses are found, paying for them is the next struggle.

Even with a discounted rate, every night a nurse stays costs over $200. For a doula, families must pay this cost out-of-pocket, which is why the doula option is accessible to minor royals, the otherwise wealthy, and the double mortgaged. If and only if the health provider is really a licensed nurse and not merely a postpartum doula, private health insurance sometimes will pick up some of this cost, especially when the baby requires oxygen or has a heart monitor.

My excellent health insurance did indeed list home-based nursing care as a benefit, but I was surprised to learn, with significant limitations. Reimbursement was capped at $80 per night, and a maximum of a handful of nights would be covered. Any amount was, of course, a help, but it still would not make night nurses doable for any significant time. I correctly predicted my health insurer's attitude toward my questions about exceptions to the limits. No information was provided about how I could get more home-based support; I needed to gut it out, like every other mother had done from time immemorial. If my babies were returned to the NICU, that was on me.

Barely seek but sometimes ye shall find. The answers walked through my front door in a stunning display of DC service efficiency. Through its Strong Start program, the District of Columbia assesses the developmental delay of every premature baby in the city. A multidisciplinary team of a speech-language pathologist, occupational therapist, physical therapist, child development specialist, and two interns showed up on my front porch to evaluate the twins. Suspending my disbelief that six-week-old babies could be assessed for anything at all, I let the team place my twins on the floor and hem and haw when each baby flopped on his face like a slug, too frail to move. The therapists flashed lights at the babies, clapped their hands to the left and to the right, and made faces and bubbles at them. An hour later, the team pronounced that each twin would have thrice-weekly therapy to strengthen his core muscles, assist his swallowing, and teach him to turn his head. Sessions would begin in a week.

As they said their goodbyes, one of the team, a very tall, very wide, middle-aged infant speech pathologist, asked, "Is there anything else we could do to support you?" I showed him my nursing order and my ever-mounting night nursing bills and asked if he had any ideas. "Apply for Medicaid," said the giant in my living room.

Laughable. We were standing in a single-family home owned by two employed adults. Medicaid is the US health program for the poor, and it was most evident that we did not and should not qualify. "Use Katie Beckett," he said. "Look it up."

Medicaid participation and billing are the stuff from which legal careers are made. The rules are complex and arcane, the qualifications to participate differ from state to state, the paperwork is legion, and the bureaucracy, formidable. I knew the barest minimum about Medicaid for adults from working in an AIDS clinic while in law school. How to get babies signed up for Medicaid, I hadn't the foggiest idea. By now, though, I had become the paperwork and bureaucracy maven. There was no system that, if I poked at it long enough, I could not defeat.

I went in search of whoever Katie Beckett was, the person who would pay for my children's night nurses. Once, she was a four-month-old baby who was partially paralyzed by viral infection. Katie passed away in 2012 and is now the patron saint of home care. Her legacy is the Katie Beckett Waiver, which Ronald Reagan, of all people, signed into law so that little Katie, who could not breathe without ventilator support, could receive institutional-level care paid for by Medicaid at home. The old Medicaid rules would have made Katie ineligible for aid if her middle-class parents removed her from the hospital, but hospitalized care cost Medicaid six times as much as home care.[8] Reagan directed his secretary of health and human services to waive the Medicaid rules for children like Katie to be treated with less expensive, home-based care rather than remaining in the hospital.

From a policy perspective, President Reagan was more concerned about cutting Medicaid's costs and, eventually, its budget. The Great Communicator employed Katie's story as an example of expensive governmental regulation that was fleecing the American taxpayer and harming children. Congress was convinced to change the allocations to Medicaid. The Katie Beckett Waiver, codified in the less friendly–sounding Tax Equity and Fiscal Responsibility Act (TEFRA), suspends the parental income requirement for the child's Medicaid coverage if the child could receive health services at home rather than in an institution. Only the child's own income is considered for Medicaid eligibility. The child, disabled and formerly hospitalized, has no job or assets and easily meets the waiver's income requirements of being far below the poverty line.[9]

Our doctor's nursing care order combined with the hospital's NICU re-admission threat made Declan and Frankie medically eligible for the waiver. To stay at home and not in the NICU, the twins had to gain weight and remain infection free to avoid exacerbating their underlying cardiovascular, respiratory, and neurological complications of TTTS. The keys to meeting these goals were specialty formulas, antibiotics, iron supplementation, and medicines, all administered on a strict timetable, morning and night. Both babies were bundled in swaddling and hats in the sweltering DC summer heat to prevent them from expending energy shivering. Declan had to be kept at an angle so he would not regurgitate his food. Each twin had congenital muscular torticollis, with neck muscles too tight for them to turn their heads. Declan's torticollis was so pronounced he had developed plagiocephaly: his head was flattened from always lying in one direction. Doctors predicted that these conditions would persist for more than twelve months but could be treated at home with some extra support. And home-based nursing care for the twins would be thousands of dollars per day less expensive than if they received the same treatment in the NICU.

As stipulated by the waiver, the twins' income—not mine—determined their eligibility for Medicaid. Lazy babies, they didn't work and had no salaries. After the extensive documentation required to demonstrate medical eligibility for the waiver, showing the twins met the poverty qualification was as easy as ticking a few boxes.

Even if qualified to receive Medicaid through the Katie Beckett Waiver, the child is not guaranteed to receive a cent for reimbursement of her medical bills. Whether services or funds are available through the waiver depends on where you live, the extent to which your state has expanded access to Medicaid, and the number of Medicaid dollars your state has managed to squirrel away. All states, except for Tennessee, have increased disabled children's Medicaid eligibility through the Katie Beckett Waiver or a similar program.[10] Yet federal pecuniary miserliness in the funds actually available through Medicaid has led fourteen states to institute waiting lists for children deemed eligible and needing services through the waiver.[11]

The District of Columbia is one of the most generous in the services it covers through the waiver and Medicaid for sick, special needs children, and it has no wait for these services. As a result, over half of DC children with special healthcare needs receive public health assistance. Across the street in Maryland, the situation is quite the opposite, with under a quarter of disabled children receiving Medicaid or similar governmental health insurance.[12]

Serendipitously, we had moved from Maryland to DC four days before the twins were born. Although many DC children receive Medicaid, few DC residents apply for and receive the waiver. This fact is both a testament to the many resources theoretically available in DC and an indictment: the city has a high rate of poverty and a low overall level of education and literacy. Those otherwise eligible cannot navigate the waiver application process, which appears to have been made deliberately onerous to discourage families from trying.[13]

Typical for Katie Beckett Waiver recipients, the twins had private health insurance through my employer. Medicaid provided "wrap-around coverage" for medically necessary services my health insurance would not cover or for costs that exceeded my health insurance plan's maximum. Medicaid also picked up other costs my health insurance denied: a helmet to reform Declan's flat head and, for his persistent anemia, pungent, high-iron formula that sold for $60 a can.

The twins' salvation, my sanity, and my spouse's night's sleep were thanks to public assistance. The American and the District of Columbia taxpayers paid not only for my children's essential healthcare but also for the convenience of night nurses. The public Strong Start program provided three years of every sort of therapy to improve my children's development, all absolutely for free. I was able to receive this assistance, while others could not, because of my ability to navigate the systems to apply and demonstrate eligibility for it and because of my luck of living in a jurisdiction where it was available. Forevermore, when a politician speaks of people on public welfare, he will be speaking of me: a woman with several children whose care she could not afford, sucking at the taxpayer's teat.

The ethics of my family's taking public funds tortured me. Unlike the majority of the 6.1 million children with special healthcare needs,[14] our family's resources far exceeded the federal poverty line. We could have obtained a second mortgage on our house or tried to pay for the twins' nurses using our credit cards—because, unlike the poor or those driven into bankruptcy by medical bills, we had banks willing to extend us credit and collateral we could draw on. Was it wrong to avoid poverty ourselves by using governmental resources intended for the impoverished? Of greater concern, were Medicaid funds the fixed pie politicians make them appear to be in the annual debate about cutting the budget for Medicaid? Would my twins' using a rules waiver to obtain Medicaid funding limit the services or money available to another child, one who was objectively more disabled and less fortunate than my children? And what of the propriety of using the Katie Beckett Waiver? For all the sympathy due to Katie Beckett and her family, the waiver was a political gambit devised by a Republican president I despised to bleed dry Medicaid and to siphon its resources from lower income minority families, disproportionately its primary users, to Republican supporters, who were white and middle class.[15]

I brought these questions to the DC Department of Health Care Finance, an entity unused to engaging in philosophical debate with callers. Sometimes, though, things work well in this city. A few transfers brought me to a manager, who listened to my angst and told me, "Ma'am, your children qualified to receive this assistance. Take it."

The funds made available through the waiver are use it or lose it; whatever remains unused in the state's coffers at the end of the fiscal year must be returned to the federal government.[16] If my twins were eligible, awarding them Medicaid benefits would not take these resources from another needy child. It would just mean that DC would return a few thousand dollars less to the federal government for redistribution to other states and initiatives. And, as a DC resident friend put it, she would rather her taxes go for the support and care of disabled children—even the slightly disabled children of a rather well-to-do family—than to a myriad of other governmental priorities about which she had not been consulted and would oppose.

An unanticipated benefit of Mary and her night nurses was a line on a source of donor breast milk for Declan. Many years before having children, and before I had any personal experience in the matter, I had been a lactation consultant in Central Asia.[17] My experiences of helping poor women conserve their resources through breastfeeding left me with a deep opposition to feeding babies artificial formula and made me a card-carrying member of the "breast is best" movement.

Yes, I was "that woman," the lactating Karen.[18] The one who glared at bottle-feeding mothers from across the restaurant while muttering under my breath. I had helped enact breastfeeding protections into law, for heaven's sake. Obamacare, for which I advocated in Congress and at the White House, made health insurance plans cover the costs of renting or purchasing a breast pump and receiving lactation consulting. Obamacare also required many employers to provide nursing parents break time and a secure location to express breast milk.[19]

Any backsliding on the commitment to breastfeed would seem to me a betrayal of the cause. Although by then pregnant with the twins, I had nursed my first child until he turned two. Even that was too little by my family's superlactating standards. My sisters and my in-laws nursed their babies on demand for at least three years and wondered at my cruelty for cutting short my child's access to liquid gold.

When I wheeled myself in to visit the twins for the first time in the NICU and found them both hooked up to feeding tubes connected to formula cans, I was very unhappy. Pissed even. No one had bothered to ask my permission before giving my babies artificial milk. Grabbing a harried NICU nurse, I demanded to know how the twins could receive some of the hospital's limited supply of donor breast milk until my personal supply ramped up enough to feed them. There was permission to give and a form to sign. The default was formula; breast milk was opt-in only.

Surely, with all the lactation-inducing herbal tea, cookies, and supplements I was taking, my milk would soon come in abundance. With my first child, I was a prizewinning dairy cow. After fully feeding my baby, I still produced so much milk that my freezer was filled to bursting with little, frozen yellow baggies, each carefully labeled with the date of extraction (and, oddly, my child's name, as if there would be some confusion as for whom these baggies were intended). I donated those baggies to at least three other babies. When my friend in California adopted an infant, I overnight shipped her hundreds of ounces of milk packed in a cooler of dry ice I finagled from a liquor store.

Quickly, I was humbled. The twins needed more and better milk than I could provide. I nursed them whenever they demanded and until they were satiated, but they remained so tiny, and Declan, so anemic. Their pediatrician instructed me to supplement Declan's nursing with bottles of formula, made double strength to increase its caloric and iron potency. But Declan broke out in eczema, itchy red patches all over his little body, a likely allergic reaction to the formula. Changing the formula type from cow-milk-based to soy had no effect except that each variant was more expensive and smelled more like paint thinner than the last.

I waded into the unregulated world of American milk sharing. Neither DC nor Maryland has a human milk bank, where donated breast milk is collected and pasteurized for distribution.[20] Out of a hospitalized setting, parents in my area must arrange for informal sharing of breast milk. There are no local or federal rules that prohibit or promote breast milk exchanges, so hungry babies find willing breast milk donors through the intermediation of Facebook.

Two milk sharing sites dominate the local breast milk grey market: Eats on Feets and Human Milk 4 Human Babies. Once you complete a questionnaire about your smoking, alcohol consumption, and other habits and tick a box pledging to tell the truth about your risk factors, you are granted access to a closed Facebook group with nonstop alerts:

> Hello fellow moms. I'm in desperate need of donated milk for my 7-month-old. He never latched well and lost 12% of his birth weight.
>
> Hi! I have several gallons of pumped milk in my deep freezer from May through September. I don't need it since I'm home to feed my baby.

Et voila! Demand meets supply, and only the transportation needs to be arranged. No one will blink an eye at a demand that the milk come from a pet-free home or that a donating mother be completely alcohol abstinent; these are reasonable requests. But if you are taking the invaluable bodily fluids of another human being for your offspring's consumption, milk sharing etiquette demands that you also offer to replace the plastic freezer baggies in which the milk is donated. Milk sharing depends on good will and trust, and in the absence of money, good manners is a stand-in currency.

Driving all over three states to retrieve breast milk from strangers was, by far, the biggest drawback of milk sharing. Picking up a hundred ounces here and a hundred ounces there made for too much work and driving when trying to keep up with the milk consumption of twins. For the more risk averse, there are greater epidemiological concerns. Informal donation networks of breast milk have no way of guaranteeing the safety of the milk exchanged or of pasteurizing it. FDA recommends against feeding your baby breast milk acquired directly from individuals or through the internet.[21] My presumption, however, was whatever is good enough for another woman's baby is good enough for mine. But others have greater fear of their baby's infection from contaminated milk, which is why milk banking and milk sharing remain far outside the mainstream in the United States.

As a nurse, Mary was more concerned that the milk we fed Declan was reliably safe and clean rather than whether it was convenient. She regarded with disdain the acrid-smelling formula that turned my sweet baby into a ruby-scaled lizard. Hitting on a solution, she suggested to me that I use her own niece's milk. Her relative had a baby who was a year older than the twins and a freezer packed with unused breast milk. She knew her niece to be healthy and her milk to be fattening.

One morning, I opened my freezer to find it stuffed full of new baggies of yellow milk, each carefully labeled with the date of expression and another baby's name. (Apparently, all mothers do this.) Declan gulped down the extra breast milk, finding it much tastier than the formula. His eczema resolved, and slowly, slowly, during the course of two years, the dots we plotted on graph paper for his age-for-weight crept up, finally appearing on an appropriate growth curve. So it came to pass that my American twins, having been guided into existence by Turkish and Venezuelan doctors who were informed by Belgian science, were nursed with Ghanaian breast milk administered by a pan-African team of nurses before being entrusted to a Salvadoran nanny and coached by DC's finest therapists.

(*Chapter Eleven*)

Facts vs. Belief

With difficult pregnancies, life-and-death decisions must be based on the information at hand, not on what future studies might show. In 2015, when I was pregnant with my twins, American hospitals would permit only conservative management and close monitoring of Stage I twin-to-twin transfusion syndrome to avoid unnecessary interventions.[1] The same approach—monitoring with no intervention—was applied to pregnancies complicated by selective intrauterine growth restriction. As for the combination of the both early TTTS and sIUGR, again, the hospitals would not permit a surgical resolution, although all agreed that each condition confounded effective treatment of the other.

The cramped view of surgery simply was the presumption of the time. Of the options of laser surgery, cord coagulation, amnioreduction, or ongoing monitoring, no proposed TTTS or sIUGR solution was supported by reliable data from a randomized controlled trial. The treatment a patient received depended on where she sought help, the laws of the jurisdiction, the beliefs held by the surgeons at that location, and what the hospitals permitted their surgeons to do.

"Expectant management," or watching the pregnancy carefully but doing nothing to intervene in it, was the most common global strategy to address early TTTS. By the mid-2000s, however, European hospitals were more likely than US hospitals to permit laser surgery for women in special circumstances.[2] For pregnant women living more than two hundred miles from a hospital offering laser surgery, having severe symptoms of uncomfortable uterine distension or a cervical length of less than fifteen millimeters, European maternal-fetal health centers would change from their default recommendations of expectant management to a prescription of laser surgery to treat TTTS.

Hospitals in the United States, however, reflexively required early TTTS to be managed by expectant management. If a patient cited her special circumstances and appealed a denial of laser surgery, American hospitals changed their recommended course of action to amnioreduction. The suggestion that patients manage their TTTS by serial removal of amniotic fluid was unique to the United States and rather out of step with the times. Even by the early 2000s, amnioreduction had fallen out of favor in Europe and the rest of the world as a treatment approach for TTTS.[3]

If we are honest, we should accept that umbilical cord coagulation may be the surest way to guarantee that a complicated mono-di twin pregnancy results in the birth of a healthy baby. Cord coagulation is a selective reduction, sacrificing the less healthy twin to save the stronger twin. The procedure requires fetoscopic surgery, posing the same surgical risks, such as infection and blood loss, to the mother as any other operation using a fetoscope. But electing to reduce the pregnancy to one baby achieves between an 80 and 93 percent survival rate for the remaining twin.[4] The now singleton is almost always born at term, thereby avoiding the risks attendant to prematurity.[5] Local and national laws may prohibit parents and doctors from choosing this option, however. Cord coagulation is most effectively done either at twenty or twenty-eight weeks of gestation,[6] thereby making it a late-term abortion according to the definitions in many countries and in several states. Although selective termination prevents the harms caused by twin pregnancy, miscarriage, and preterm birth to both mother and baby, policymakers have deemed it to be an unacceptable treatment for TTTS and sIUGR.

With cord coagulation taken off the table, an international evidence base was building that laser surgery was the next best course to achieve the birth of at least one physically and neurologically sound baby. The aptly named Eurofetus trial from 2004 had demonstrated the clear superiority of laser ablation over amnioreduction for managing TTTS in general.[7] These findings were confirmed in a 2013 study, which found overall survival of the twins to be about the same with laser surgery and conservative management but worse for amnioreduction.[8] Given that the majority of TTTS expectant management cases worsened, the North American Fetal Therapy Network therefore opined that only laser surgery protected a Stage I pregnancy against double fetal loss or very preterm delivery before twenty-six weeks.[9]

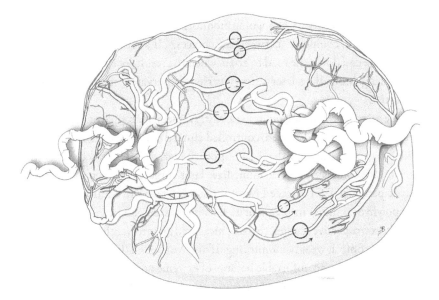

Connecting blood vessels across the amnions. From L. Van Der Veeken, I. Couck, J. Van Der Merwe, L. De Catte, R. Devlieger, J. Deprest, and L. Lewi, "Laser for Twin-to-Twin Transfusion Syndrome: A Guide for Endoscopic Surgeons," *Facts, Views and Vision in Obstetrics and Gynecology* (September 2019): 197–205, 198, fig. 2, https://www.ncbi.nlm .nih.gov/pmc/articles/PMC7020942/. Image reproduced with permission from UZ Leuven (www.uzleuven.be).

A long-awaited meta-analysis, a study of studies, of TTTS interventions was published in 2016. It found that more babies survive when laser surgery is used as a first-line treatment for Stage I TTTS, instead of taking a wait-and-see approach of expectant management.[10] Laser ablation is the best form of treatment for TTTS even when TTTS is diagnosed before sixteen weeks, as mine was, or after twenty-six weeks.[11]

These results are not strong, however, given the few pregnancies studies and the difficulty of conducting a controlled trial. The findings may also be tainted with bias, as they are derived from observational data with all its challenges of confusing cause and effect and explaining rare events.[12] The 2016 study concluded that it could not judge how best to achieve the survival of both twins and their mother in a pregnancy like mine. As for managing Stage I

TTTS with laser surgery or ongoing monitoring, the study's authors professed themselves "in equipoise" between the choices.[13] If anything, the 2016 study kicked the can down the road to 2020, when the results of a randomized trial comparing immediate laser surgery versus conservative management were expected.

The 2020 study turned out to be a bust. A research group from Paris began an international, randomized, controlled clinical TTTS Stage I trial in 2010. The intent was to answer the big question: for early TTTS, which was better, conservative management or immediate laser surgery?[14] Patients who could participate had TTTS Stage I (within the more restrictive European criteria for polyhydramnios) in pregnancies between sixteen and twenty-six weeks. Unlike retrospective studies, this one measured an intervention, laser surgery, against a control, weekly monitoring. If any woman's TTTS worsened, or if she became very uncomfortable because of extreme uterine growth from over-inflated amniotic sacs or due shortening, she was cleared for laser surgery. The goal was to achieve the survival of both twins until six months after birth.[15] Unfortunately, this study was closed in 2019 because few patients joined it. The world of TTTS survivors and patients waited for the publication of some analysis of the study participants. But as of the writing of this book in 2021, these results have yet to be released.

As for TTTS complicated by sIUGR, in 2015, there was not even a globally agreed-on definition of what constituted sIUGR, even as it was used as the reason to deny me laser surgery to resolve my twins' TTTS. The best advice the Society for Maternal-Fetal Medicine could offer was that a TTTS pregnancy complicated by sIUGR receive "frequent, e.g., twice weekly" Doppler scans of the umbilical artery's blood flow once the twins reached viability.[16]

If 2020 failed to bring results about early TTTS, at least the annus horribilus[17] offered some advancement in understanding sIUGR. Consensus was achieved in defining sIUGR. According to the new, agreed-upon definition, and similar to TTTS, sIUGR is also staged according to its severity. It can involve an estimated fetal weight of one twin below the third percentile or a combination of factors: when one twin is estimated to weigh below the tenth percentile, the weights between the twins differ by 25 percent or more, or the blood circulation between the smaller fetus and the placenta is impeded.[18] With my smaller twin below the third percentile for estimated fetal weight and with one twin presumed to weigh between 30 and 50 percent more than the other, I easily met this new definition.

The good news is that at least one twin survives in almost 90 percent of sIUGR cases. The bad news is overall survival drops to 65 percent when TTTS confounds sIUGR.[19] The ugliness is that sIUGR is different enough from TTTS and other complications of an identical twin pregnancy that the optimal treatment for one may be the least desirable intervention for the other.[20]

The 2020 sIUGR study included a table of three instances when laser surgery had been used to manage a sIUGR pregnancy—too few examples from which conclusions could be drawn.[21] Another recent but very limited study showed that laser surgery intervention on sIUGR twins "bordering on TTTS" resulted in more fetal deaths than expectant monitoring, the watching and waiting approach I ultimately took.[22] But, in a result that would have gutted me, more babies born alive in the expectant monitoring died within their first six months of life.[23]

Hoping for answers may be a fool's errand, but pregnant women cannot find any actionable guidance from study findings that shrug at doing nothing versus doing everything. Given the very narrow window for decision-making during pregnancy, there may be a cost to waiting to perform surgery on a Stage I TTTS pregnancy too. Postponing laser surgery to separate twins' connected blood vessels potentially could increase the risk of one twin's dying and the surviving twin's being exposed to hemorrhagic brain injury and resulting neurological damage. Miscarriage of one twin increases the likelihood that the amniotic sacs will rupture prematurely and that the mother will have a very preterm birth.[24] Premature birth is a significant danger for a TTTS-surviving twin, putting the baby at risk for later sickness and death.

Studies that focus only on improving survival miss the point. Compared to severe TTTS, which is almost always fatal, early TTTS usually remains stable enough that doctors can monitor the pregnancy and induce birth before both twins deteriorate in utero. Ensuring live births through expectant management, however, does not account for pregnancies that progress to severe TTTS and require laser surgery or that end in miscarriage or preterm birth with neurological impairment.[25]

For any hope of a TTTS pregnancy ending with live and neurologically healthy infants, what mothers and doctors need is information about which course of action—laser surgery, expectant management, or something else—leads to the best long-term outcome for surviving children. At age two, TTTS survivors treated with laser surgery had a 9 percent incidence of severe neurological disability. Five percent of these toddlers had cerebral palsy.[26] The harm of a difficult pregnancy is incredibly long lasting: lower declarative memory scores are seen in twelve-year-olds who suffered poor blood circulation from the placenta while they still were forming inside their mothers.[27]

A more recent and much larger clinical trial repeated earlier findings on the extent of severe neurological disability and pessimistically found that, although more TTTS babies are surviving to childbirth, "improvement in outcome of TTTS has reached a plateau."[28] Over the past decade, the very best medicine has not improved neurological disease–free survival after laser treatment for TTTS. And no study yet has published clear comparisons of long-term neurological outcomes of TTTS survivors who did not undergo fetal surgery with those who did.

The only true advance in TTTS care in the five years since I was pregnant has been in the surgical technique to be used—if, in fact, surgery is chosen as the TTTS management strategy. The Solomon technique, in which an equator line is burnt around the entirety of the twins' shared placenta, has been shown to be too much, the surgical equivalent of using a bazooka to kill a mosquito. Instead, the better approach is a "partial Solomon," where the surgeon lasers a semicircle only where anastomoses lead from one amniotic sac to the other. Lasering should not be done where no blood vessels are seen because doing so more commonly leads to placental abruption, in which the placenta separates prematurely from the uterine wall, resulting in sudden hemorrhaging.[29] The placenta is thought to be thinner or weaker where it does not have visible blood vessels, and burning it with a laser causes damage that could result in preterm birth.

My race against time to have TTTS surgery may have been a bit contrived. Whereas in 2015, laser surgery had to be completed in a narrow window between 16 to 26 weeks of gestation, there is some evidence that laser treatment in TTTS before 16 and after 26 weeks is feasible, safe, and may improve outcomes immediately before and after birth.[30] My TTTS progressed steadily through my pregnancy with my donor twin deteriorating rapidly, but the one surgeon willing to operate on me moved to Europe when I was around

19 weeks. Children who received in-utero laser surgery after 26 weeks show better neonatal outcomes than those who had TTTS but who did not receive surgery. A pregnancy remains 40 weeks and most twins are still born before being full-term. The deadline for laser surgery may now have stretched, although only slightly.

Significant questions remain about how to treat TTTS, especially TTTS that remains at the "early" state or is confounded with sIUGR. Much evidence links a child's fetal growth restriction to the child's poor cognitive performance, probably because sIUGR babies are usually born prematurely with low birth weight.[31] Likewise, TTTS babies are almost universally premature. It may be prematurity and resulting low birth weight, and not TTTS, that causes so much neurological damage to these children. Premature babies are more likely to suffer cerebral injuries at birth, culminating in cerebral palsy. Although the greatest damage is found in the most premature babies, late-preterm infants, born from thirty-four to thirty-six weeks, still face tough odds for escaping unscathed from an early birth. It is likely that these still preterm babies will have moderate neurodevelopmental delay.[32]

Thirty percent of TTTS survivors have mild cerebral palsy and other neurological or cognitive disability. Even minor disability has a major effect on children's educational and social attainment. The greatest improvement in long-term outcomes for TTTS babies could be found in a TTTS treatment that does not result in premature birth, as both fetal surgery and expectant management do. A noninvasive treatment, such as high-intensity focused ultrasound to sever conjoined anastomoses, could stop the transfusion of one twin by the other and prevent puncturing the amniotic sac and sending the mother into preterm labor.[33]

Another small gift from the years that have passed since my twin birth is a revision of the thirty-seven-year-old study on using cerclage to prevent premature twin birth.[34] For the entirety of my own life, cerclage was presumed to be of no help to a woman trying to stave off preterm birth of her twins. For however effaced, shortened, or dilated her cervix, stitching it shut seemed ineffective in keeping her twins inside of her. Finally, there is hope, where before there was none. A randomized controlled study—a good one!—showed cervical cerclage for women with dilated cervixes in their second trimester reduced preterm birth and associated infant mortality in twin pregnancies.[35]

The positive effect of cerclage for twin pregnancies was so strong, reducing preterm birth by more than 50 percent at less than twenty-eight weeks, that the study was stopped midway through so the intervention could be offered to the control group. There might be a way to stave off the ravages of prematurity for TTTS twins.

But nothing is ever clear with TTTS. Other scientists have cast doubt on the theory that it is prematurity that causes so much damage to babies who survive TTTS. A study of every TTTS pregnancy in the Netherlands discovered that more than half of the babies with severe neurological disease were born at more than thirty-two weeks and were not, by definition, extremely premature. Neither had these babies suffered a cerebral injury. Something else related to TTTS, perhaps the imbalance of blood between them, the anemia the donor suffers, or the excess of blood inflating the recipient, harmed these children.[36] What is really scary is that no one knows when this damage occurs or whether whatever is dangerous about TTTS persists after birth. In a conclusion that makes any parent's blood run cold, the Dutch TTTS researchers said, "Our data show the importance of assuring long-term follow-up for all TTTS survivors at least until school age, regardless of their gestational age at birth or the presence of severe cerebral injury on ultrasound scans."[37]

We are left with trying to answer one final question my doctors could not. My pregnancy never fully matched the TTTS criteria because, at its nadir, the donor fetus's amniotic fluid pocket remained .2 centimeters deeper than that required for TTTS. The hospital ethics boards therefore regarded me as having sIUGR only, although my doctors clinically diagnosed me as having Stage I TTTS. For my doctors' proposed laser ablation treatment to be approved, we needed to point to evidence of the long-term neurological benefit to the twins of laser surgery for sIUGR. All eyes turned to studies in Europe that we hoped would have the answer, but my pregnancy progressed faster than did the science.

The intervening years have provided only a little clarity on this issue. An analysis of all available studies of sIUGR interventions since 2004 (comprising twenty-one retrospective and thirteen prospective cohort studies, three noncomparative studies, one cross-sectional study, and, significantly, only one case-controlled study) found six that reported on cognitive health of children who were treated for sIUGR before birth.[38] Of these, two studies were large enough, involving 48[39] and 217[40] children, to try to draw some conclusions about which sIUGR treatment provided the best long-term protection for children's neurological health. And yet, no. Equating these two studies is comparing apples to oranges. The studies' reporting on neurological outcomes was so inconsistent that neither doctors nor patients can determine which sIUGR intervention results in the least neurological morbidity.[41]

One of the doctors I consulted during my pregnancy published results that proclaim that sIUGR "patients treated with laser therapy are likely to have an improved neurological outcome over those managed expectantly."[42] No difference was found after age two in the personal–social, adaptive, motor, communication, and cognitive development of children born of sIUGR pregnancies that were treated either with expectant management or laser therapy. The researchers surmise that the laser-treated group eventually will be found to have improved neurodevelopmental outcomes because children in this group were born at significantly older gestational ages.

This was the information we were all seeking! But a glance at the study's sample size makes the public health expert in me know that a pregnant woman could not place all her hope in these results. Even more so than TTTS, sIUGR in twin pregnancies remains a rare, fatal, and poorly understood condition with few surviving children to study over the years. A mere fourteen children in the laser therapy group were compared with six children in the expectant management group, limiting any conclusions that could be drawn about the long-term neurological outcomes of laser treatment for sIUGR.[43]

With all this focus on the fetuses, one would think that they were the patients the doctors were so invested in studying and saving. But the fetuses have no life without their mother, and it is she who has sought care for her pregnancy. In the reams of studies I found both during and after my twin pregnancy, there was hardly a mention of the subject of all these studies: the pregnant woman.[44] She was merely the vessel that contained a complicated research problem. A plethora of sources describe the harm of untreated TTTS on the mother: hypertension and stroke, preeclampsia, hemorrhage, kidney and liver failure. The effect of sIUGR on the pregnant woman are less documented but also include preeclampsia and high blood pressure.[45] The risks, to the woman, of not resolving TTTS or sIUGR presumptively are the drawbacks, to the woman, of expectant management of TTTS or sIUGR.

Nevertheless, these are not presented as a rationale for choosing to intervene in the pregnancy. Conversely, the immediate or long-term harm to the woman of conducting fetoscopic surgery is not commonly provided as a reason for not pursuing laser coagulation of her fetuses' connecting blood vessels.

The consequences of obstetrical interventions for a woman are so unimportant as to not warrant study or discussion. The first systematic review to evaluate safety reporting in *any* obstetric trials (in that case, for preeclampsia medicines) was in 2017. Randomized trials on pregnancy interventions collect an enormous amount of data about fetuses and children born, including mortality, significant disability, and birth defects. The review's authors gallantly "encouraged" other researchers to consider women as humans with worth beyond their gestating function and to report adverse outcomes to women of the interventions studied.[46]

Tellingly, the one mention of the paucity of studies on maternal health following fetoscopy for sIUGR as compared to fetoscopy for TTTS suggests the need for reporting on procedural complications and maternal outcomes that, presumably, would affect her current pregnancy.[47] Adverse outcomes on women's health are those that are independent of her pregnancy. These could include a woman's pain during laser surgery or afterward. Any scarring to her abdomen. The long-term effect on her cervix or uterus. The consequences for her mental health. Whether her future fertility, reproductive health, or sexual health could suffer. In 2015, these issues had not been studied, so no one could judge the effect on women of choosing the state-of-the-art therapy for their fetuses.

Then and now, the attitude of most doctors, scientists, and hospitals is "baby or bust." For the many studies that now exist of TTTS and sIUGR, I struggled to find out about the effect on the woman of interventions into her body on behalf of her twin pregnancy. Even as the science has evolved to save the lives of identical twins, women have been forgotten. It took until 2019 for researchers to note this informational lack, calling it "disappointing."[48]

With "baby or bust," it is the woman who sometimes bursts, occasionally physically and, other times, mentally. Now we know for fetoscopic fetal surgery, the severe complication rate is approximately 2 percent and the minor complication rate 4 percent.[49] Severe complications include those that could kill or permanently maim the mother: heart attacks, lung collapses, hysterectomies, and sepsis. Poor outcomes that are bad but not bad enough to kill the mother were judged to be minor. Such minor inconveniences of fetoscopic laser surgery include the mother's hemorrhaging more than one liter of blood, which is significant enough to require transfusions.[50]

These surgical complications are nothing to shrug at, but they are, blessedly, rare. Deeply concerning is the finding that, over the long term, a whopping one out of three women who undergo fetoscopic surgery experience psychological symptoms.[51] Some studies show that up to 65 percent of women suffer an adverse psychological outcome after laser surgery,[52] especially when surgery is accompanied with the loss of one of the twin fetuses.[53] But what these psychological issues are, and the extent to which other factors were controlled, is not described.

The poor and variable reporting of laser surgery procedural complications and maternal outcomes in both TTTS and sIUGR studies of interventions is not just saddening; it is unsafe and unethical. Laser surgery is increasingly being offered to women pregnant with twins to the supposed benefit of their fetuses. Because it offers no direct medical benefit to the mother, from an ethical perspective, maternal risks should be minor and acceptable to her.[54] Ethics also requires that these risks are explained to the woman and that she agrees to assuming them.[55] Without being aware of the risks this intervention poses to themselves, women cannot properly give informed consent to fetoscopic laser treatment. Women also must be supported in comparing the risks of intervention with the risks of only monitoring the pregnancy's natural evolution. Biomedical ethics obligates medical providers to respect women's autonomy by clarifying for them the health risks that are independent from those to their fetuses and deferring to women should they choose to prioritize diminishing their own risks at the expense of their fetuses.[56]

In my case, and although they thought differently at the time, my doctors now agree that laser surgery would have been the wrong choice to make. The donor twin pumped away all his blood to his twin and received in return very little oxygenated and food-nourished blood through his two-vessel, poorly implanted, umbilical cord. He survived only because of the blood transfused to him through the blood vessels connected to his twin. Using laser ablation to sever those connecting blood vessels would have cut the smaller twin's lifeline.

Expectantly managing my pregnancy turned out to be determinative: it told me when I needed to give birth. Using a Doppler ultrasound and a computerized heart scan, the doctors monitor the blood flow to and from the babies' hearts and brains to establish the best timing for delivery, which is the moment when either twin looks as if it will die if it stays in the mother, but both twins seem big and healthy enough to be born.[57] My doctor said he had gotten this calculus correct with Declan. He was born just in time; any longer inside of me, and he likely would have been a stillbirth. And a stillbirth that late in the pregnancy would have killed Frankie, too.

By preventing the laser surgery I requested, the IRBs at Johns Hopkins and in Miami ensured the live birth of both my twins, who survived the neonatal period, did not show severe neurological morbidity by age two, and are still alive today. I too survived pregnancy and childbirth with little damage beyond persistent hemorrhoids, diastasis recti, core muscular weakness, and a tanked career. The American taxpayers and my employer's health insurance plan picked up the over one-million-dollar price tag for the twins' and my medical care, cushioning the financial pummeling of a high-risk childbirth and lengthy NICU stay. My fight to save all of us did not drive my family into poverty.

But this happy ending was not achieved because the IRBs correctly read the nascent data about survival rates and longer-term neurological health for both twins. The data about laser surgery in cases like mine was not available when the IRBs blocked me from receiving the care I desired and my doctors recommended. Instead, these results were achieved by ignoring my informed and considered wishes and the then best practice proposed by my experienced and expert doctors. Antiabortion bias was, as my doctors suspected, the most likely reason for the IRBs' substitution of their judgment for my own and that of my personal surgeons.

We reach the end of my story, and I am left to wonder whether the ends justified these means. As it happened, my twins and I are very lucky to emerge mostly unscathed from TTTS and sIUGR; only my rights and opinions were trammeled. But the outcome could have easily gone the other way, and that would have made for a harder balance of the tradeoffs of my choices for the dictates of national or hospital politics. What if one twin died or was permanently neurologically impaired? What if I had died? What if my family had gone bankrupt from the medical costs of saving the twins? My great fear is that someone reads my story, thinks, "it all turned out well," concluding that women's rights matter not and using these pages to justify further restrictions on women's maternal and reproductive health treatment options.

I was viscerally offended that the hospitals' model was to restrict my decision-making power while ensuring I assumed all legal, financial, and reputational risk for my pregnancy's outcome. As an attorney, I understand the hospitals' position; risk shifting is the art of good contract writing and the key to preventing—or winning—litigation. As the patient being served by the healthcare system, I view this strategy as violating the obligation to respect my autonomy. When it comes to twins, there is a scarcity of quality data available to guide the evidence-based obstetrician.[58] Shady sales pitches from device and drug companies' promotional material may influence doctors' decision-making. Not every doctor is swayed by the latest study published in a medical journal, and it takes years for medical practice to integrate research findings.

For this lack of evidence, how best to proceed was ultimately a competition of beliefs: mine and my doctors' against the hospitals'. Less deference was given to my opinions and research, which lost the wrestling competition against the heavyweight hospitals. As a public health professional, I know that shared decision-making between provider and patient is incredibly important. Yet there was no sharing the medical decisions about my body and my children and no recognition of the damage done by ignoring the patient's will. When she is not heard, the patient will be less likely to comply with doctors and hospitals' guidance for her care in the future, wondering whether their advice is factual or only a statement of faith or morals.

Politicians in most states and the majority of justices on the US Supreme Court also would substitute their judgment for women's when it comes to pregnancy and maternal health. Recently passed laws prohibit doctors from using safer gynecological procedures in favor of more risky ones. Or the law orders doctors to inflict harm on their patients by, for example, requiring that ectopic pregnancies are reimplanted from the fallopian tubes to the uterus.[59] Other laws criminalize abortions even when the fetus would be born without a brain or heart or when the birth would injure the mother.[60] If a patient asks her health insurer, physician's practice, or pharmacist about her options for contraception, pregnancy intervention, or obstetrics, there is no legal obligation for them to provide accurate information or any information at all.[61] The pregnant person bears the entire burden of her pregnancy, and whether she can influence the outcome of that pregnancy is increasingly determined by privilege, especially race, wealth, and education, not by medicine and science.

It is fair to probe my assumption that, had the doctors and the politicians let me make my own decisions regarding my pregnancy, arming myself with all these data would have altered my decision-making. Most pregnancy and parenting choices make not an iota of sense, which is why the experts refuse to defer to parents' crazy beliefs. You have unprotected sex, convinced you won't get pregnant. You drink just a little wine, justifying it as under the amount that would cause fetal damage. You continue the pregnancy when you know you cannot care for or afford the child to be produced. You spend a million dollars to save your baby and then risk his life in a crib with a cute bumper that matches your nursery decor.[62] You bring children into this world with the destruction of the planet's climate nevertheless impending. You oppose abortion, although you may one day need to terminate a pregnancy to save yourself.

Knowing the facts and the science does not change our actions; we just pray that the likely and foreseeable outcome will not befall us. I sought talismanic protection in trusting I would defy the odds. Beyond overresearching and worrying to death every issue, thus resulting in this book, I did little to bend the arc of outcomes toward a different conclusion.

This same inertia born of optimism is what explains parents' fierce dedication to inclined baby sleepers, their well-publicized linkage with infant deaths notwithstanding. Inclined sleepers, such as the Fisher-Price Rock 'n Play, were on the market for only ten years, from 2009 to 2019, when the US Consumer Product Safety Commission (CPSC) backed their recall and all major vendors pulled the sleepers from their internet and brick-and-mortar stores. In that short time, these products killed seventy-three babies and had over a thousand reported, near-miss incidents.[63] Yet parents continue to buy inclined sleepers on the secondhand market and childcare providers persist in using them, insisting they are the next best thing to sliced bread.[64] The cult of the inclined sleeper perseveres even through death: devotees argue the data are all wrong; it's a personal choice to put your own baby at risk; and an attentive parent will be able to save her baby from any harm.[65] For these parents' beliefs in their own superpowers, infants are the sacrificial lambs.

After the NICU saved them, I brought my tiny, not-even-four-pound babies home from the hospital—and installed them in the matching, inclined sleepers that constituted the bulk of my living room furniture. For a change of scenery, I would move the twins from these to hanging basinets, which swung from a fixed frame like hammocks, and then back to the expensive, automated inclined sleepers we controlled with our iPhones. If mechanized swaying and bouncing in the electronic sleepers was too much, we could go low-tech and put the babies in floor-level, vibrating inclined sleepers that we bounced with our feet. So constantly were the twins in inclined sleepers that the cradles' tinny soundtrack of EDM-infused lullabies still plays on a loop in my head.

I knew the risks, even if I did not fully appreciate them. Since 2012, pediatrics blogs had reported babies' deaths suspected to be tied to inclined sleepers, and authorities in Australia, Canada, and the United Kingdom banned the products from being sold as sleepers in those countries. By 2015, when the twins were born, US concern had grown so pitched that safety standards were established for infant-inclined sleep products. But these standards were wholly voluntary and were based in politics, not science. Child safety advocates vociferously opposed the new standards, arguing online and in court that US regulators should have never allowed inclined sleepers on the market.[66]

A sleep-deprived, musically assaulted brain plays tricks on you, rationalizing the irrational. I believed, incorrectly and against evidence, that the only way to stop the chorus of wailing and for Declan not to regurgitate his milk was to keep the twins constantly at the ten- to thirty-degree angle inclined sleepers provided. This deadly incline did nothing to improve acid reflux, which pediatricians have long known. Instead, it offered a smorgasbord of ways to die.[67] The slanted position was optimal for causing babies' heads to slump forward, crushing their tracheas, and blocking their airflow. The sleepers' slope made it possible that the twins would roll over and suffocate on the sleeper's sidewalls or headrest. As my babies did multiple times, the babies could slide down the sleeper and crumple into a pile at its base, again posing risk of asphyxiation. Or the child could become tangled in the sleepers' restraints and hang itself. But while the twins lived, their inclined sleepers ensured they slept, meaning that I could work, sleep, and parent my other child.

It took until the end of 2019 for the CPSC to harden its mealy-mouthed warnings against inclined sleepers and to state, clearly, "These products do not provide a safe sleep environment."[68] But still the US government did not undertake a mandatory recall of inclined sleepers, allowing manufacturers to remove their products from the market voluntarily and leisurely. By late 2020, companies were still recalling inclined infant sleepers, and thousands of new and used sleepers still circulated in the market.[69] Before I was aware of their recall, I handed down my multiple inclined sleepers to my sisters for use with my nieces and nephews. And they passed the sleepers on to their friends for their babies. Everyone raves at how well their babies sleep in these devices. No one has died, yet.

Irrational fealty to a belief—even in the face of death—could also describe political convictions. After spending hundreds of pages arguing that lives are saved through empowering individual reproductive and maternal healthcare choices and providing a compelling story to prove my point, I will bet I have changed no minds on abortion. Those who were favorably inclined to permit women to choose to intervene in their pregnancies still are prochoice, while those whose religions or political parties already proscribe abortion remain antiabortion.

There are "four factors that determine whether we are going to change our beliefs—our old belief, our confidence in that old belief, the new piece of data, and our confidence in that piece of data."[70] The further away the data are from what you already believe, the less likely it is that you will change your belief. The innate psychological process of confirmation bias makes us accept data that confirm our existing convictions and to disregard data that do not conform to what we already believe. When encountering facts that do not match our beliefs, we try to reframe those facts by discrediting them. We decide those facts do not fit the narrative we have constructed for ourselves and are therefore not good evidence of the phenomenon being debated.[71]

Those rejecting out-of-hand the evidence presented here will do so because it is mentally uncomfortable to hold simultaneously contradictory ideas or values. This discomfort, or cognitive dissonance, is triggered by a situation in which a person's belief clashes with new evidence introduced to that person.[72] For those morally opposed to abortion, holding onto that belief and accepting my story will cause psychological unease. Reducing cognitive dissonance would require changing your mind, but confirmation bias indicates that it would be easier to discount the data.

If my twin story and the studies are accurate, perhaps your antiabortion beliefs are wrong. To hold on to these beliefs would indicate you are comfortable with an outcome where one or both twins died, where both twins were born severely neurologically impaired, where I died leaving my toddler motherless, or where all three of us, the twins and I, died. Alternatively, if you think your antiabortion beliefs are absolutely correct, then my stories and the studies must be false or irrelevant. Your view is that it would be better to let all pregnancies take their course, no matter the long odds for a successful outcome or the consequences of how many survive the pregnancy or the quality of life of the survivors. After all, my twins and I somehow rolled triple snake eyes in a game of almost no chances. If you prize nonintervention over all else, I ask, would you choose the likely and grim results of my pregnancy for yourself? For your daughter? Or is the most "prolife" course of action to gamble and shoot the moon?

When everyone else around you is deeply opposed to permitting individuals to make their own reproductive decisions, there is little chance of your accepting my story as a reason to change your political views and voting behavior. To change would move you out of step with your peers and community. There could be a real social cost to rethinking your views on abortion and maternal healthcare; those around you could ridicule or condemn you. On issues for which the social value of our beliefs matters a lot, it can be much harder to change our minds.[73]

The only approach that is said to challenge beliefs successfully is the one I have employed here: explaining, in much detail, the effect of implementing antiabortion policies and bias.[74] When approached with storytelling accompanying scientific facts, even those opposed to a different point of view moderated their disagreement. Their contrary arguments became less intense, and their attitudes began to change. Rather than beating people over their heads with polemics, situating facts within a larger narrative makes those facts more memorable and accessible. Walking through the implications of how science affects politics and the even greater effect of politics on the science of twin pregnancy and maternity could stimulate thinking that, ultimately, will result in more positive outcomes for all those who are surprised by a rare and complicated health crisis.[75]

Beliefs are what we would will to happen, all evidence and experience notwithstanding. Acting from a position of privilege, able to obtain almost any desired information, and equipped with the education to understand the data collected, throughout my twin pregnancy and afterward, I still fell sway to magical thinking disguised as hope. The statistics showed an infinitesimally small possibility that my pregnancy would end well, with the twins and me healthy and intact. The greater indications were that things would go badly for one, two, or all three of us. Instead of being proactive and doing absolutely everything to change the equation in my favor, especially when faced with overwhelming resistance, it was far easier to resort to wishing all would be fine.

When the chips were down, I did not fly to Belgium for a fetoscopic surgery prohibited in the United States. After seeking the very best medical advice available, I encountered too many barriers to capitalize on this advice. Instead, I tried unproven and discredited therapies, like lying in extended bedrest and drinking protein shakes, offered by unlicensed and unregulated practitioners, under the pretense that doing a small bit of something was better than doing absolutely nothing. I also prayed, although I doubted God's influence on nature's biological processes and have since lost my faith. Mostly, I simply kept plodding forward, day after day, and the wheel of fortune eventually turned in my favor. After all, each believes she is the exception to every rule devised by science or by man, and if fate so decrees, luck will smile on us.

Epilogue

At five years old, Frankie and Declan are healthy, happy little boys. They do not have significant or even moderate neurological, intellectual, or cognitive disabilities. Their fine and gross motor development is slightly slower than their peers', but they continue to progress, almost meeting the milestones for their age.

The hole in Frankie's heart closed. He had continual respiratory infections for his first two years, perhaps related to the respiratory distress he experienced at birth or his short time on the ventilator in the NICU. For him, we continually replenished our supply of bubblegum pink amoxicillin in the refrigerator. Frankie also had trouble swallowing and speaking, his food and words sliding from his lips without control. Occupational and speech therapy, paid for by the US taxpayers through Strong Start, fixed both.

Declan's aortic coarctation also resolved miraculously without surgery. His tethered spinal cord has also not required surgical intervention, and he does not have spina bifida or paralysis of the lower limbs. He also does not have a tail, but his favorite animals are monkeys; perhaps he intuits a commonality with them. Several other surgeries corrected his small developmental issues caused by prematurity, including bilateral inguinal hernias. These operations and the many IVs from the NICU left still-visible scars all over Declan's body, especially on his wrists and feet. His fight to gain weight continues, with chronic acid reflux blocking his food absorption during much of his early life. Thanks, however, to a year of donor breast milk from our night nurse and four years of nutritional supplementation with Pediasure (and, around the winter holidays, eggnog), Declan's height is not stunted.

With the twins' histories of neurological, cardiac, and respiratory problems and given their propensity for infection that has required years of antibiotics, the encroaching plague of the novel coronavirus was deeply frightening.

COVID-19 involves systemic attacks on brains, hearts, and lungs.[1] Although children are supposed to suffer less than adults, should the twins become infected, I presumed the coronavirus would do them terrible harm and fell them quickly.

We locked ourselves in our house for nine months, leaving only for outdoor, socially distanced, masked activities. COVID entered anyway and infected us the same week the FDA approved the first vaccines for emergency use. Our nanny attended church services, was infected, and brought the infection home to us and to her own family. We all tested positive with the strange (and, certainly, erroneous) exception of Declan, who sleeps in the same bed and had the same symptoms as positive Frankie.

Surprisingly, the twins sailed through their coronavirus infections with little more than the typical symptoms of any childhood virus: runny noses, congestion, headaches, some appetite loss, and bad tempers. Our lengthy quarantine was punctuated by drawn-out battles over toys and TV time. Both twins broke out in full-body rashes and Frankie had swollen, blistered "COVID toes." But that was it; the twins' older siblings (I adopted another child in 2020) and the adults in the house, myself included in their number, suffered much more. The twins may have avoided the dreaded multisystem inflammatory syndrome in children (MIS-C) associated with COVID-19.[2] I am watching them carefully and hoping fate, the less generous sister of luck, spares them once more.

The twins are mindful of my exhortations to control the spread of COVID by maintaining hygiene and washing hands. Declan recently informed me that he was sucking on a hard candy as he was sitting on the potty. The candy fell from his mouth and into the toilet bowl. He fished the candy out and prudently washed it and his hands before popping the sweet back into his mouth to enjoy. Again, he suffered no ill effect. His immune system is heartier than we could have ever imagined a few years ago.

As is true for many donor TTTS twins, Declan struggles more than Frankie, the TTTS recipient. Declan is shorter and does not resemble his identical twin at all. Though, in a reversal of the typical confusion of not being able to tell twins apart, it's only everyone else who cannot mistake Frankie for Declan; the twins themselves believe they look exactly alike. When Declan was tiny, he would identify his own reflection as "Frankie." To make up for the nutrition he pilfered from Declan while in the womb, Frankie today saves parts of his meals for Declan, tossing him pizza and buttered breadcrusts from across the table. Betwixt the two of them, they lick the platters clean.

The effects of TTTS and sIUGR linger, though. They are subtle, perceived by my mother's eye, if not by anyone else. Growth and development assessments do not capture the extent of Declan's challenges, although, based on the Ages and Stages Questionnaire we complete each year, his doctors assure me that he is completely normal. But Declan loses his balance often, tripping over his own two feet. He has fallen so frequently that he required three root canals by age four for shattered teeth. Eventually, his front tooth had to be extracted, which, when combined with a perpetual bump on his head, string-bean stature, and Barack Obama ears, give Declan a forlorn look. Potty training, even by kindergarten, is an on-going project, yet to be mastered. Holding a pencil, recognizing or writing letters, and reading are elusive skills. For now, Declan likes to cuddle next to Frankie, who turns the pages of books for him and tells him stories.

My workplace situation never really improved after having the twins, although it was not impeded by them. It was, perhaps, thorny from the start. Two weeks before the twins' surprise premature birth, my organization changed its policies to shorten the maternity leave it offered. I hoped to be grandfathered in under the old rules; yet, alas, I was not. Instead, the human resources department told me to get a doctor's note saying I was sick, so I could go onto short-term disability and stay out of work for longer. My doctor was unwilling to lie for my job convenience.

I was not more ill than the typical postpartum woman who had suffered an emergency C-section and hemorrhage. The American system does not recognize the woman's need to recuperate from childbirth, and one out of every four American women returns to work within ten days of giving birth.[3] Nor does the American system, government-provided or private insurance–covered, pay for postpartum mothers to recover.

The United States is unique among industrialized nations in this lack of respect for birth parents and lack of appreciation of their recuperation needs. In France, mothers' pelvic floor physical therapy is paid out of the public purse. The French consider vaginal "reeducation" an essential part of postpartum care, and obstetricians routinely prescribe ten to twenty sessions for each woman at her eight-week postnatal checkup.[4] As a result, even French women who have had multiple children can jump on trampolines without becoming incontinent. The moms in my exercise classes could only dream of staying dry while leaping or running.

My babies needed my dedicated care, but a doctor's note for them would not apply to me, and the time off I had received exceeded the minimum legal requirements for family and medical leave, had these applied to me.[5] Out of time and energy to fight, I did as my job coach had instructed: I took the full component of maternity leave available to me and burned my banked annual leave to stay home with the twins for just short of six months. When I returned, I worked shortened workweeks for the next eighteen months to breastfeed the twins and tend to them.[6] I then finagled a transfer to another agency within the same system of organizations. Finally, after eleven years and three biological children, I managed to overcome the harm maternity had done to my career and have just won my first raise and promotion. Of course, the men who began working at the same place at the same time are now one and two levels above me in the organization; one is my boss. They also took little or no parental leave after the births of their children, so they did not disrupt their professional progression.

During these years of focus on the twins, Declan and Frankie's older brother began to display wanton oppositional behavior. My spouse and I attended parenting classes, which said we were the likely cause, as we had failed to spend enough quality "special time" with our eldest child and had disrupted his life by having twins. Later, our firstborn was diagnosed with autism spectrum disorder (ASD). Addressing and treating autism has made for its own struggle and my rapid education about the world of 504 plans, individualized education plans, and the school politics that accompany them. Autism's cause is unknown, but our poor parenting is not to blame. Research shows that, like schizophrenia,[7] ASD is associated with an older father.[8]

There is something to nature's imperative to bear children in your twenties and thirties. Not only does the mother lessen her chances of having fraternal twins and a difficult pregnancy, but the father also reduces the likelihood of creating his offspring from gametes that are past their prime. With every year that a man ages, he accumulates, on average, two new mutations in the DNA of his sperm.[9] These disruptions in developing sperm might be a precursor to aberrant embryonic and placental development.[10] Babies of older fathers are at increased risk for low birth weight, seizures, and the need for ventilation immediately after birth. Men who were forty-five or older were 14 percent more likely to have a child born prematurely, and men fifty or older were 28 percent more likely to have a child that required admission to the neonatal intensive care unit.[11] Older fathers too are suspected of being responsible for placental problems in their pregnant partners, although no one has yet studied whether an older father is responsible for the root causes of sIUGR.[12]

A younger parent too has more energy and, arguably, more patience for his children.[13] Having been single until his early forties and having embarked on childbearing around the time his peers' children were leaving for college, my spouse had difficulty making the transition to fatherhood. Kindergarten, especially virtual, bilingual kindergarten using Zoom, directed by the parents, has been his Waterloo. During our coronavirus debacle, when the municipal authorities quarantined our entire family at home, we were left without childcare but needing to work full-time and simultaneously monitor our children's schooling. My spouse was to superintend the twins' online classes for a morning while I attended an online staff meeting. Yes, the classes are in Spanish at our children's immersion school, but I thought he could hack it, even if he didn't speak the language. Our home is typically loud, echoing with the noisy exclamations of four children. Presuming it was emanating from one of the kids, I ignored the screaming downstairs so I could concentrate on my job. By 10:00 a.m., three parents of other kindergarteners texted me to complain that my spouse's shouting was disturbing the class and that he should "take a breath." The twins were running through the house a few minutes later, my spouse having lost patience entirely with online schooling and declaring a recess for the rest of the day.

On the plus side of the older father ledger, childbearing later in life has certain advantages for both parent and child. Older parents have more established careers with financial security and the flexibility to reduce their working hours, work at home, or schedule their workdays to better suit their personal and family needs.[14] They report being more emotionally prepared to have children and committed to developing positive relationships with their coparent and with the rest of their family. Compared to children of younger fathers, male children with fathers of "advanced paternal age" have higher IQs, stronger focus on academic subjects of interest, and social aloofness.[15]

These traits combine to convey an advantage for modern life and translate into future higher socioeconomic status. In other words, an older father has had more time to build a successful life for himself, and his children, too, have a better-than-even chance to be successes in school, work, and life.

I barely made the temporal cut-off for children, and my spouse far exceeded his sell-by date. Despite these many concerns competing for my attention and my advanced age, I still wanted to have another child. I've found that I love small children, especially my own, and although I may be mediocre as a professional, I am adept at caring for babies. I adopted a refugee, adding a teenage girl to our passel of little boys and immersing me in the political fights about immigration and separated refugee families. But a teen lacks that intoxicating new baby smell and has needs far more complex than nursing and diapering.

Having barely survived three babies in two years, my spouse is absolutely opposed to gestating another infant or, should lightning strike us twice, twins. I cannot convince him otherwise. We have given away our triple stroller and all the tiny, outgrown baby shoes.

(*Notes*)

Introduction

1. See Daniel Cox, "Abortion May Be Mobilizing More Democratic Voters Than Republicans Now," FiveThirtyEight, October 31, 2018, https://fivethirtyeight .com/features/abortion-may-be-mobilizing-more-democratic-voters-than -republicans-now/.

Chapter One

1. See WebMD, "Blighted Ovum," Grow, https://www.webmd.com/baby/blighted -ovum#1.

2. See World Health Organization (WHO), "Maternal Mortality," Fact Sheets, September 19, 2019, https://www.who.int/news-room/fact-sheets/detail/maternal -mortality.

3. See Nicholas J. Kassebaum et al., "Global, Regional, and National Levels of Maternal Mortality, 1990–2015: A Systematic Analysis for the Global Burden of Disease Study 2015," *Lancet* 388 (October 2016): 1775–1812, Findings section, https://www.sciencedirect.com/science/article/pii/S0140673616314702.

4. The racial disparity of these data is staggering. Black women die at many times the rate of white women, with the maternal mortality rate for non-Hispanic Black women at 37.3 compared to 14.9 for non-Hispanic whites. See Centers for Disease Control and Prevention (CDC), National Center for Health Statistics, "Key Findings," November 9, 2020, https://www.cdc.gov/nchs/maternal -mortality/index.htm.

5. See Nina Martin and Renee Montagne, "U.S. Has the Worst Rate of Maternal Deaths in the Developed World," National Public Radio (NPR) and ProPublica Special Series, Lost Mothers: Maternal Mortality in the U.S., May 12, 2017, https://www.npr.org/2017/05/12/528098789/u-s-has-the-worst-rate-of-maternal -deaths-in-the-developed-world.

6. See WHO, "The Right to Health," https://www.ohchr.org/Documents/Issues /ESCR/Health/RightToHealthWHOFS2.pdf.

7. See William C. Shiel Jr., "Medical Definition of the Standard of Care," MedicineNet, December 21, 2018, https://www.medicinenet.com/script/main/art.asp?articlekey=33263.

8. See Guttmacher Institute, "Contraceptive Use in the United States by Demographics, May 2021, https://www.guttmacher.org/fact-sheet/contraceptive-use-united-states (citing 2018 population estimate).

9. According to my gynecologist, most doctors try to avoid sharp (metal) curettage with pregnancy D&C. Instead, physicians often use a plastic curette that is attached to a suction device.

10. See Lindsey Lanquist, "A New Arkansas Abortion Law Basically Bans Second Trimester Abortions," *Self,* February 3, 2017, https://www.self.com/story/arkansas-trap-law.

11. See Guttmacher Institute, "Bans on Specific Abortion Methods Used after the First Trimester," June 1, 2021, https://www.guttmacher.org/state-policy/explore/bans-specific-abortion-methods-used-after-first-trimester.

12. Ibid.

13. See Mara Gordon, "The Scarcity of Abortion Training in America's Medical Schools," *Atlantic,* June 9, 2015, https://www.theatlantic.com/health/archive/2015/06/learning-abortion-in-medical-school/395075/.

14. FDA, "Misoprostol (Marketed as Cytotec) Information," Postmarket Drug Safety Information for Patients and Providers, July 10, 2015, https://www.fda.gov/drugs/postmarket-drug-safety-information-patients-and-providers/misoprostol-marketed-cytotec-information.

15. See Jennifer H. Tang, Monica Dragoman, João Paulo Souza, and Nathalie Kapp, "WHO Recommendations for Misoprostol Use for Obstetric and Gynecologic Indications," *International Journal of Gynecology and Obstetrics* 121 (February 2013): 186–89, https://www.researchgate.net/publication/235715137_WHO_recommendations_for_misoprostol_use_for_obstetric_and_gynecologic_indications.

16. See ACOG, "Induction of Labor," *ACOG Practice Bulletin* 107 (August 2009), https://www.mnhospitals.org/Portals/0/Documents/patientsafety/Perinatal/acog--practice_bulletin_107_2009.pdf.

17. See Olga Khazan, "When Abortion Is Illegal, Women Rarely Die. But They Still Suffer," *Atlantic,* October 11, 2018, https://www.theatlantic.com/health/archive/2018/10/how-many-women-die-illegal-abortions/572638/.

18. See Julia Belluz, "Abortions by Mail: The FDA Is Going after Online Pill Providers," Vox, March 12, 2019, https://www.vox.com/2019/3/12/18260699/misoprostol-mifepristone-medical-abortion.

19. See Ushma D. Upadhyay, Sheila Desai, Vera Zlidar, Tracy A. Weitz, Daniel Grossman, Patricia Anderson, and Diana Taylor, "Incidence of Emergency Department Visits and Complications after Abortion," *Obstetric Gynecology* 125 (January 2015): 175–83, Results section (on medication abortions), https://pubmed.ncbi.nlm.nih.gov/25560122/.

20. See Sarah Christopherson, "It's Time to #MailTheAbortionPill," National Women's Health Network, July 1, 2020, https://www.nwhn.org/its-time-to-mailtheabortionpill/.

21. See American College of Obstetricians and Gynecologists v. U.S. Food and Drug Administration, Civil Action No. TDC-20-1320 (D. Md. Jul. 13, 2020), https://www.acog.org/-/media/project/acog/acogorg/files/advocacy/pi-order-medication-abortion-71320.pdf.

22. See Carrie N. Baker, "The Abortion Pill Mifepristone Just Became Easier to Get," *Ms.*, July 21, 2020, https://msmagazine.com/2020/07/21/the-abortion-pill-mifepristone-just-became-easier-to-get/.

23. See U.S. Food and Drug Administration v. American College of Obstetricians and Gynecologists, 592 U.S. ____ (2020) (Alito, J., dissenting).

24. COVID infections were absolutely not on the downswing when the federal government submitted its brief. See Johns Hopkins University, "Confirmed COVID19 United States Cases by County," for September–October 2020, https://coronavirus.jhu.edu/us-map.

25. See Anna North, "What Amy Coney Barrett on the Supreme Court Means for Abortion Rights," Vox, October 26, 2020, https://www.vox.com/21456044/amy-coney-barrett-supreme-court-roe-abortion.

26. See Caroline Kelly, "Federal Court Upholds Block on In-Person Medication Abortion Requirements," CNN, December 9, 2020, https://www.cnn.com/2020/12/09/politics/court-upholds-medication-abortion-supreme-court/index.html.

27. See U.S. Food and Drug Administration v. American College of Obstetricians and Gynecologists, 592 U.S. ____ (2021) (Roberts, C. J., concurring), https://www.supremecourt.gov/opinions/20pdf/20a34_3f14.pdf.

Chapter Two

1. See Carla Ransom, "The Management of Monochorionic-Diamniotic Twins," presented at the High-Risk Conference, Vanderbilt University, November 30, 2020, slide 8, https://studylib.net/doc/18119470/the-management-of-monochorionic-diamniotic-twins.

2. See Nora Caplan-Bricker, "For the First Time Ever, Thirty-Something Women

Are Having More Babies Than Their Twenty-Something Counterparts," *Slate*, May 17, 2017, https://slate.com/human-interest/2017/05/cdc-data-says-women-in-their-thirties-are-having-more-babies-than-women-in-their-twenties.html.

3. See Quoctrung Bui and Claire Cain Miller, "The Age That Women Have Babies: How a Gap Divides America," *New York Times*, August 4, 2018, https://www.nytimes.com/interactive/2018/08/04/upshot/up-birth-age-gap.html.

4. For 2013 data, see Joyce A. Martin, Brady E. Hamilton, Michelle J. K. Osterman, Anne K. Driscoll, and T. J. Mathews, "Births: Final Data for 2015," *National Vital Statistics Report* 66, no. 1 (January 5, 2017): 1–69, 13, https://www.cdc.gov/nchs/data/nvsr/nvsr66/nvsr66_01.pdf. For 2018 data, see Centers for Disease Control and Prevention, *National Data, Assisted Reproductive Technology (ART) Data* (2018), https://nccd.cdc.gov/drh_art/rdPage.aspx?rdReport=DRH_ART.ClinicInfo&rdRequestForward=True&ClinicId=9999&ShowNational=1.

5. See M. I. Evans, S. Andriole, and D. W. Britt, "Fetal Reduction: 25 Years' Experience," *Fetal Diagnosis and Therapy* 35 (2014): 69–82, The Problem section, https://www.karger.com/Article/FullText/357974.

6. Although one study found a higher likelihood (1.45 percent) of monozygotic twins following ART, provided good quality embryos were cultured together for a longer period of time (3.5 days). See Huihui Wang, Haibo Liu, Weijia Chen, Yuan Sun, and Yuewei Li, "Identifying Risk Factors Related to Monozygotic Twins after Assisted Reproductive Technologies," *European Journal of Obstetrics and Gynecology* 230 (2018): 130–35, Conclusions section, https://doi.org/10.1016/j.ejogrb.2018.09.004.

7. See Iva Skoch, "Wanderlust: Bride Kidnapping in Kyrgyzstan," *The World*, Public Radio International, October 12, 2010, https://www.pri.org/stories/2010-10-12/wanderlust-bride-kidnapping-kyrgyzstan.

8. See Mark I. Evans and David W. Britt, "Multifetal Pregnancy Reduction," Global Library of Women's Medicine (May 2009), https://www.glowm.com/section-view/heading/multifetal-pregnancy-reduction/item/214# (under review as of June 2021).

9. See ACOG, "Multifetal Pregnancy Reduction," Committee Opinion no. 719 (September 2017): 2, https://www.acog.org/Clinical-Guidance-and-Publications/Committee-Opinions/Committee-on-Ethics/Multifetal-Pregnancy-Reduction.

10. Ibid.

11. Ibid.

12. See Associated Press, "'Octomom's' Doctor Apologizes for Implanting 12 Embryos," CBSN Bay Area, October 21, 2010, https://sanfrancisco.cbslocal.com/2010/10/21/octomoms-doctor-apologizes-for-implanting-12-embryos/.

13. See Evans and Britt, "Multifetal Pregnancy Reduction."

14. See John Morrison, "Twin Gestation and Premature Birth," *Journal of Perinatology* 25 (2005): 1–3, https://www.nature.com/articles/7211224. More recent and verified cost data are hard to locate. Gianna Melillo, in "How Much Does It Cost to Give Birth in the United States? It Depends on the State," *American Journal of Managed Care*, May 15, 2020, https://www.ajmc.com/view/how-much-does-it-cost-to-give-birth-in-the-united-states-it-depends-on-the-state, reports average vaginal birth costs for a single baby of $8,300 in Arkansas and more than double that, $20,000, in New York.

15. See Jonathan Muraskas, and Kayhan Parsi, "The Cost of Saving the Tiniest Lives: NICUs versus Prevention," *Virtual Mentor* 10 (2008): 655–58, https://journalof ethics.ama-assn.org/article/cost-saving-tiniest-lives-nicus-versus-prevention /2008-10.

16. See ACOG, "Multifetal Pregnancy Reduction," 2–3.

17. See Carla Ransom, "The Management of Monochorionic-Diamniotic Twins," slide 19.

18. See Traci B. Fox, "Multiple Pregnancies: Determining Chorionicity and Amnionicity," Thomas Jefferson University, Department of Radiologic Sciences Faculty Papers (2006), paper 1, 2, https://jdc.jefferson.edu/rsfp/1.

Chapter Three

1. See Bhaskar Chakravorti, "The Case against Big Tech's Election Strategies," *Foreign Policy*, October 20, 2020, https://foreignpolicy.com/2020/10/20/the -case-against-big-techs-election-strategies/.

2. See Yatan Pal Singh Balhara, "Indexed Journal: What Does It Mean?," *Lung India* 29, no. 2 (April–June 2012): 193, https://www.ncbi.nlm.nih.gov/pmc /articles/PMC3354504/.

3. See C. J. Mann, "Observational Research Methods. Research Design II: Cohort, Cross Sectional, and Case-control Studies," *Emergency Medicine* 20, no. 1 (2003): 54–60, https://emj.bmj.com/content/20/1/54.

4. L. Van Der Veeken, I. Couck, J. Van Der Merwe, L. De Catte, R. Devlieger, J. Deprest, and L. Lewi, "Laser for Twin-to-Twin Transfusion Syndrome: A Guide for Endoscopic Surgeons," *Facts, Views and Vision in ObGyn* 11, no. 3 (September 2019): 197–205, 197, https://www.ncbi.nlm.nih.gov/pmc/articles /PMC7020942/.

5. Lisa E. Moore, "Twin-to-Twin Transfusion Syndrome," Medscape, April 2, 2020, Background section, https://emedicine.medscape.com/article/271752-overview#a6.

6. See Rúben A. Quintero, Walter J. Morales, Mary H. Allen, Patricia Bornick,

Patricia K. Johnson, and Michael Kurger, "Staging of Twin-Twin Transfusion Syndrome," *Journal of Perinatology* 19, no. 8, pt. 1 (2000): 550–55, https://www .researchgate.net/publication/12668082_Staging_of_Twin-Twin_Transfusion _Syndrome.

7. See Lynn L. Simpson, "Twin-Twin Transfusion Syndrome," Society for Maternal-Fetal Medicine (SMFM) Clinical Guideline, *American Journal of Obstetrics and Gynecology* (January 2103): 3–18, https://www.ajog.org/article/S0002 -9378(12)01980-1/pdf.

8. See Van Der Veeken et al., "Laser for Twin-to-Twin Transfusion Syndrome," 198.

9. Ibid., citing L. Lewi, "Monochorionic Diamniotic Twin Pregnancies Pregnancy Outcome, Risk Stratification and Lessons Learnt from Placental Examination," *Verhandelingen—Koniklijke Academie voor Geneeskunde van Belgie* 72, nos. 1–2 (2010): 5–15, https://pubmed.ncbi.nlm.nih.gov/20726437/.

10. See Van Der Veeken et al., "Laser for Twin-to-Twin Transfusion Syndrome," 198.

11. The Twin to Twin Transfusion Syndrome (TTTS) Foundation, https://web .archive.org/web/20200922233534/http://www.tttsfoundation.org/help_during _pregnancy/summary.php ("The outlook for twins with TTTS was hopeless over 20 years ago, but now we have the ability to diagnose the condition early (with ultrasound scans) and implement treatments that will ultimately lead to most of the twins surviving and being healthy").

12. Marjolijn S. Spruijt, Enrico Lopriore, Sylke J. Steggerda, Femke Slaghekke, and Jeanine M. M. van Klink, "Twin-Twin Transfusion Syndrome in the Era of Feto-scopic Laser Surgery: Antenatal Management, Neonatal Outcome and Beyond," *Expert Review of Hematology* 13, no. 3 (2020): 259–67, 259, https://www .tandfonline.com/doi/full/10.1080/17474086.2020.1720643.

13. See Mater Mothers' Hospital, "Twin to Twin Transfusion Syndrome," http:// brochures.mater.org.au/brochures/mater-mothers-hospital/twin-to-twin -transfusion-syndrome.

14. Ibid. See also Catherine Barrea, Christian Debauche, Olivia Williams, Stéphanie Jasienski, Patricia Steenhaut, Thierry Sluysmans, Pierre Barnard, and Corinne Hubinont, "Twin-to-Twin Transfusion Syndrome: Perinatal Outcome and Recipient Heart Disease according to Treatment Strategy," *Journal of Paediatrics and Child Health* 49, no. 1 (2013): e28–34, e28, https://pubmed.ncbi.nlm.nih .gov/23279102/, noting 57% neonatal mortality following amnioreduction. See also Laurent J. Salomon, Lisa Örqvist, Philippe Aegerter, Laurence Bussieres, Sté-phane Staracci, Julien J. Stirnemann, Mohammad Essaoui, Jean-Pierre Bernard,

and Yves Ville, "Long-Term Developmental Follow-Up of Infants Who Partici-pated in a Randomized Clinical Trial of Amniocentesis vs. Laser Photocoagula-tion for the Treatment of Twin-to-Twin Transfusion Syndrome," *American Jour-nal of Obstetrics and Gynecology* 203 (2010): 444.e1–7, Results section, https://www.ajog.org/article/S0002-9378(10)01109-9/fulltext, finding 61% mortality and 17% neurological impairment with amnioreduction.

15. See Spruijt et al., "Twin-Twin Transfusion Syndrome in the Era of Fetoscopic Laser Surgery."

16. See Femke Slaghekke et al., "Fetoscopic Laser Coagulation of the Vascular Equa-tor versus Selective Coagulation for Twin-to-Twin Transfusion Syndrome: An Open-Label Randomized Controlled Trial," *Lancet* 383 (2014): 2144–51, https://pubmed.ncbi.nlm.nih.gov/24613024/. See also Jeanine M. M. van Klink et al., "Neurodevelopmental Outcome at 2 Years in Twin-Twin Transfusion Syndrome Survivors Randomized for the Solomon Trial," *American Journal of Obstetrics and Gynecology* 214, no. 1 (January 2016): 113.e1–7, Results section, https://pubmed.ncbi.nlm.nih.gov/26297943/.

17. See Sprujit et al., "Twin-Twin Transfusion Syndrome in the Era of Fetoscopic Laser Surgery."

18. See J. Stirnemann, G. Chalouhi, M. Essaoui, N. Bahl-Buisson, P. Sonigo, A-E Millischer, A. Lapillonne, V. Guigue, L. J. Salomon, and Y. Ville, "Fetal Brain Imaging following Laser Surgery in Twin-to-Twin Surgery," *British Journal of Obstetrics and Gynecology* 125, no. 9 (August 2016): 1186–91, 1186, https://obgyn.onlinelibrary.wiley.com/doi/full/10.1111/1471-0528.14162.

19. See, e.g., Spruijt et al., "Twin-Twin Transfusion Syndrome in the Era of Feto-scopic Laser Surgery."

20. See Quintero et al., "Staging of Twin-Twin Transfusion Syndrome."

21. See Jeanine M. M. van Klink, Hendrik M. Koopman, Monique Rijken, Jo-hanna M. Middledorp, Dick Oepkes, and Enrico Lopriore, "Long-Term Neuro-developmental Outcome in Survivors of Twin-to-Twin Transfusion Syndrome," *Twin Research and Human Genetics* 19, Special Issue 3: Twin-Twin Transfusion Syndrome (June 2016): 255–61, https://www.cambridge.org/core/journals/twin-research-and-human-genetics/article/longterm-neurodevelopmental-outcome-in-survivors-of-twintotwin-transfusion-syndrome/CCBB4304CADD7700853 7967F3857027E.

22. See ClinicalTrials.gov, Study: NCT01220011, "Randomized Controlled Trial Comparing a Conservative Management and Laser Surgery (TTTS1)," https://clinicaltrials.gov/ct2/show/NCT01220011.

23. See "Chorionic Villus Sampling (CVS)," *Pregnancy, Birth and Baby*, July 2020, https://www.pregnancybirthbaby.org.au/chorionic-villus-sampling-cvs.

24. See National Health Service (UK), "Complications: Chorionic Villus Sampling," July 20, 2018, https://www.nhs.uk/conditions/chorionic-villus-sampling-cvs/risks/.

25. See Lewis B. Holmes, Marie-Noel Westgate, Hanah Nasri, and M. Hassan Toufally, "Malformations Attributed to the Process of Vascular Disruption," *Birth Defects Research* 110, no. 2 (January 2018): 98–107, 98, https://onlinelibrary.wiley.com/doi/abs/10.1002/bdr2.1160.

26. See Mayo Clinic, Amniocentesis, Patient Care and Health Information, November 12, 2020, https://www.mayoclinic.org/tests-procedures/amniocentesis/about/pac-20392914.

27. See Ronald J. Wapner, "Invasive Prenatal Diagnostic Techniques," *Seminars in Perinatology* 29, no. 6 (December 2005): 401–4, 401, https://www.sciencedirect.com/science/article/abs/pii/S0146000506000048?via%3Dihub.

28. See Francesca Malvestiti, Cristina Agrati, Beatrice Grimi, and Eva Pompilii, "Interpreting Mosaicism in Chorionic Villi: Results of a Monocentric Series of 1001 Mosaics in Chorionic Villi with Follow-Up Amniocentesis," *Prenatal Diagnosis* 35 (July 2015): 1117–27, 1117, https://www.researchgate.net/publication/280537297_Interpreting_mosaicism_in_chorionic_villi_Results_of_a_monocentric_series_of_1001_mosaics_in_chorionic_villi_with_follow-up_amniocentesis.

29. See Dartmouth-Hitchcock, *Prenatal Screening: Is It Right for You?* (2013) 16, 26, https://www.dartmouth-hitchcock.org/sites/default/files/2021-02/prenatal_testing_booklet_20121129.pdf.

30. See I. Kennerknecht, G. Barbi, M. Djalali, K. Mehnert, M. Schneider, R. Terinde, and W. Vogel, "False-Negative Findings in Chorionic Villus Sampling: An Experimental Approach and Review of the Literature," *Prenatal Diagnosis* 18 (December 1998): 1276–82, 1276, https://pubmed.ncbi.nlm.nih.gov/9885019/ (a very old source indeed).

31. See U.S. National Library Medicine, "What Is Noninvasive Prenatal Testing (NIPT) and What Disorders Can It Screen For?" MedlinePlus (November 9, 2020), https://ghr.nlm.nih.gov/primer/testing/nipt.

32. See Nuffield Council on Bioethics, "Our Concerns about Non-Invasive Prenatal Testing (NIPT) in the Private Healthcare Sector," February, 8, 2019, https://www.nuffieldbioethics.org/blog/nipt-private, describing "serious issues with how some (not all) clinics and NIPT test providers are marketing and offering NIPT in the UK," including misleading use of statistics, poor information about the

tested-for conditions, low testing accuracy for rare conditions, and poor follow-up support for families with concerning test results.

33. See FDA, "The FDA Warns against the Use of Many Genetic Tests with Unapproved Claims to Predict Patient Response to Specific Medications: FDA Safety Communication," October 31, 2018, https://www.fda.gov/medical-devices/safety-communications/fda-warns-against-use-many-genetic-tests-unapproved-claims-predict-patient-response-specific.

34. See Glee TV Show Wiki, "Finn Hudson," https://glee.fandom.com/wiki/Finn_Hudson.

35. See Social Security Administration, "Top 10 Baby Names of 2019," https://www.ssa.gov/oact/babynames.

36. See Social Security Administration, "Change in Popularity from 2018 to 2019," https://www.ssa.gov/oact/babynames/rankchange.html.

37. See Clarity Campaign Labs, "Partisan Name Calculator," https://www.claritycampaigns.com/names.

Chapter Four

1. See University of California, San Francisco, Benioff Children's Hospitals, Fetal Treatment Center, "Twin to Twin Transfusion Syndrome (TTTS)" (2013), https://fetus.ucsf.edu/ttts.

2. Asma Khalil, "Modified Diagnostic Criteria for Twin-to-Twin Transfusion Syndrome prior to 18 Weeks' Gestation: Time to Change?," *Ultrasound in Obstetrics and Gynecology* 804, February 25, 2017, https://obgyn.onlinelibrary.wiley.com/doi/full/10.1002/uog.17443, noting that TTTS diagnosis "is based on the sonographic criteria of amniotic fluid discordance: polyhydramnios in the recipient twin, with a deepest vertical pocket (DVP) ≥ 8 cm prior to twenty weeks and ≥ 10 cm after twenty weeks, and oligohydramnios in the donor twin, with a DVP ≤ 2 cm at any gestational age."

3. See F. D'Antonio, A. O. Odibo, F. Prefumo, A. Khalil, D. Buca, M. E. Flacco, M. Liberati, L. Manzoli, and G. Acharya, "Weight Discordance and Perinatal Mortality in Twin Pregnancy: Systematic Review and Meta-Analysis," *Ultrasound Obstetrics and Gynecology* 52 (July 2018): 11–23, Synthesis of the Results, https://obgyn.onlinelibrary.wiley.com/doi/full/10.1002/uog.18966.

4. See Children's Hospital of Philadelphia (CHOP), "Selective Intrauterine Growth Restriction (sIUGR)," https://www.chop.edu/conditions-diseases/selective-intrauterine-growth-restriction-sIUGR; sIUGR is also called selective fetal growth restriction (sFGR).

5. Ibid.

6. See Mostafa El-Feky and Yuranga Weerakkody, "Single Umbilical Artery," Radiopaedia, https://radiopaedia.org/articles/single-umbilical-artery.

7. See Georgios Theophilou, E. Martindale, and J. Kilner, "Correlation of Two Vessel Cords Detected on Antenatal Ultrasound Scans with Obstetric Outcomes," *Archives of Disease in Childhood—Fetal and Neonatal Edition* 95 (2010): 29–30, https://fn.bmj.com/content/95/Suppl_1/Fa29.4.

8. Cathrine Ebbing, Torvid Kiserud, Synnøve Lian Johnsen, Susanne Albrechtsen, and Svein Rasmussen, "Prevalence, Risk Factors and Outcomes of Velamentous and Marginal Cord Insertions: A Population-Based Study of 634,741 Pregnancies," *PLoS One* 8, no. 7 (July 2013), https://www.ncbi.nlm.nih.gov/pmc/articles/PMC3728211/.

9. Ibid.

10. Ibid.

11. Ibid., table 6.

12. Ibid., 1.

13. See Ramesha Papanna and Eric Bergh, "Twin-Twin Transfusion Syndrome and Twin Anemia Polycythemia Sequence: Screening, Prevalence, Pathophysiology, and Diagnosis," UpToDate, January 17, 2020, https://www.uptodate.com/contents/twin-twin-transfusion-syndrome-and-twin-anemia-polycythemia-sequence-screening-prevalence-pathophysiology-and-diagnosis.

14. See National Organization for Rare Disorders, "Spina Bifida," 2007, https://rarediseases.org/rare-diseases/spina-bifida/.

15. See Rachel Feltman, "Newborn Girl Might Have Been Carrying Her Parasitic Twins," *Washington Post*, February 11, 2015, https://www.washingtonpost.com/news/speaking-of-science/wp/2015/02/11/newborn-girl-might-have-been-carrying-her-parasitic-twins/.

16. See National Cancer Institute, "Teratoma," Dictionary of Cancer Terms, https://www.cancer.gov/publications/dictionaries/cancer-terms/def/teratoma.

17. See I. Karaman, D. Erdoğan, S. Ozalevli, A. Karaman, Y. H. Cavuşoğlu, M. K. Aslan, and O. Cakmak, "Fetus in Fetu: A Report of Two Cases," *Journal of Indian Association of Pediatric Surgery* 13, no. 1 (January 2008): 30–32, https://www.ncbi.nlm.nih.gov/pmc/articles/PMC2810823/.

18. See Maria Masters, "Vanishing Twin Syndrome," What to Expect, November 16, 2020, https://www.whattoexpect.com/pregnancy/pregnancy-health/complications/vanishing-twin-syndrome.aspx.

19. Ibid.

20. See S. Farook, R. O'Kane, and A. Tyagi, "Tale of a Human Tail: Case Report of

a Torted Human Tail," *British Journal of Neurosurgery* 22, no. 1 (2008): 135–36, https://www.tandfonline.com/doi/full/10.1080/02688690701818935?src =recsys.

Chapter Five

1. See Brown University, Alpert Medical School, "Twin to Twin Transfusion Syndrome," http://med.brown.edu/pedisurg/Fetal/FetalProgramTTTSNarrative .html.

2. See Pew Research Center, "U.S. Public Continues to Favor Legal Abortion, Oppose Overturning Roe v. Wade," August 29, 2019, https://www.pewforum .org/fact-sheet/public-opinion-on-abortion/.

3. Ibid.

4. See Emily Guskin and Scott Clement, "Abortion Support Is the Highest It's Been in Two Decades as Challenges Mount," *Washington Post*, July 10, 2019, https:// www.washingtonpost.com/politics/2019/07/10/abortion-support-is-highest-its -been-two-decades-two-decade-high-challenges-roe-mount/.

5. See Pew Research Center, "U.S. Public Continues to Favor Legal Abortion, Oppose Overturning Roe v. Wade."

6. See Guskin and Clement, "Abortion Support Is the Highest It's Been."

7. Ibid., citing an annual poll conducted by the *Washington Post* and ABC News.

8. See Gallup, "Abortion," In Depth: Topics A to Z, https://news.gallup.com/poll /1576/abortion.aspx.

9. Ibid.

10. Ibid.

11. Ibid.

12. Ibid.

13. See ObamaCareFacts.com, "ObamaCare and Women: ObamaCare Women's Health Services," August 8, 2014; updated October 1, 2018, https://obamacare facts.com/obamacare-womens-health-services/.

14. See Society for Maternal and Fetal Medicine, "Twin-Twin Transfusion Syndrome," Clinical Guidance, August 1, 2014, https://www.smfm.org/publications /80-twin-twin-transfusion-syndrome.

15. Ibid.

16. Aetna, "Fetal Surgery in Utero," *Medical Clinical Policy Bulletins*, no. 449 (May 20, 2021), http://www.aetna.com/cpb/medical/data/400_499/0449 .html#dummyLink2.

17. See Guttmacher Institute, "Regulating Insurance Coverage of Abortion," June 1,

2021, https://www.guttmacher.org/state-policy/explore/restricting-insurance
-coverage-abortion.

18. Ibid.

19. Ibid.

20. Ibid.

21. See Society for Maternal and Fetal Medicine, "Twin-Twin Transfusion Syndrome."

22. See Amy Goldstein, "Judge Blocks Trump Effort to Roll Back Birth Control Mandate Nationwide," *Washington Post*, January 14, 2019, https://www.washingtonpost.com/national/health-science/judge-blocks-trump-effort-to-roll-back-birth-control-mandate-nationwide/2019/01/14/abba97e4-181f-11e9-8813-cb9dec761e73_story.html.

23. Ibid.

24. See "Moral Exemptions and Accommodations for Coverage of Certain Preventive Services under the Affordable Care Act," *Federal Register* 83, no. 211 (November 15, 2018): 57592–631, Purpose section, https://www.federalregister.gov/documents/2018/11/15/2018-24514/moral-exemptions-and-accommodations-for-coverage-of-certain-preventive-services-under-the-affordable.

25. See Shanoor Seervai, Roosa Tikkanen, and Sara R. Collins, "Trump Administration Appeals Contraception Case to SCOTUS: What This Means for Women's Health," *To the Point* (blog), October 9, 2019, https://www.commonwealthfund.org/blog/2019/what-recent-federal-courts-rulings-contraception-mean-us-womens-health.

26. See Little Sisters of the Poor Saints Peter and Paul Home v. Pennsylvania, 140 S. Ct. 2367 (2020).

27. See Lauren Egan, "Women Rally in Support of Elizabeth Warren by Sharing Their Own Pregnancy Discrimination Stories," NBC News, October 9, 2019, https://www.nbcnews.com/politics/2020-election/women-rally-support-elizabeth-warren-sharing-their-own-pregnancy-discrimination-n1064316.

28. See General Electric v. Gilbert, 429 U.S. 125 (1976).

29. The Pregnancy Discrimination Act of 1978, 42 U.S.C. § 2000e-(k) (1976 & Supp. 1 1978), https://www.eeoc.gov/laws/statutes/pregnancy.cfm.

30. See Young v. United Parcel Service, 135 S.Ct. 1338, 1344 (2015).

31. See EEOC, "Pregnancy Discrimination Charges EEOC and FEPAs Combined: FY 1997–FY 2011," Statistics, https://www.eeoc.gov/eeoc/statistics/enforcement/pregnancy.cfm.

Chapter Six

1. See Christian Bamberg and Kurt Hecher, "Update on Twin-to-Twin Transfusion Syndrome," *Best Practice and Research: Clinical Obstetrics and Gynaecology* 58 (July 2019): 55–65, 57, https://pubmed.ncbi.nlm.nih.gov/30850326/.

2. See Simpson, "Twin-Twin Transfusion Syndrome."

3. See FDA, "Information Sheet Guidance for IRBs, Clinical Investigators, and Sponsors: Frequently Asked Questions about Medical Devices," January 2006, https://www.fda.gov/files/about%20fda/published/Frequently-Asked-Questions -About-Medical-Devices---Information-Sheet.pdf.

4. Ibid., 14.

5. See FDA, "Humanitarian Device Exemption," September 5, 2019, https://www .fda.gov/medical-devices/premarket-submissions/humanitarian-device -exemption.

6. See FDA, "Humanitarian Device Exemption (HDE) Postmarket Activities," September 5, 2019, https://www.fda.gov/medical-devices/humanitarian-device -exemption/humanitarian-device-exemption-hde-postmarket-activities.

7. See American Medical Association (AMA), "Code of Medical Ethics Opinion 1.1.3," Ethics: Patients Rights, https://www.ama-assn.org/delivering-care/ethics /patient-rights.

8. FDA, "Institutional Review Boards Frequently Asked Questions: Guidance for Institutional Review Boards and Clinical Investigators," Information Sheet, January 1998; updated September 5, 2019, https://www.fda.gov/regulatory -information/search-fda-guidance-documents/institutional-review-boards -frequently-asked-questions#GeneralQuestions.

9. FDA, "Protection of Human Subjects; Informed Consent," Final Rule, 46 FR 8942, January 27, 1981; updated April 24, 2019, https://www.fda.gov/science -research/clinical-trials-and-human-subject-protection/protection-human -subjects-informed-consent.

10. See FDA, "Pregnant Women: Scientific and Ethical Considerations for Inclusion in Clinical Trials: Guidance for Industry," Draft Guidance, Revision 1 (April 2018): 5, https://www.fda.gov/media/112195/download. See also Lynne P. Yao, Division of Pediatric and Maternal Health, Office of New Drugs, Center for Drug Evaluation and Research, FDA, "New Guidance for Industry on Pregnant Women and Risk Communication," Advisory Committee Meeting on the Pregnancy and Lactation Labeling Rule, May 14, 2018, https://www.nichd.nih.gov /sites/default/files/2018-05/03-Risk_Communication_Advisory.pdf.

11. See FDA, "Pregnant Women."

12. See Anna C. Mastroianni, Ruth Faden, and Daniel Federman, "Women and Health Research: A Report from the Institute of Medicine," *Kennedy Institute of Ethics Journal* 4, no. 1 (March 1994): 55–62, https://muse.jhu.edu/article/245708.

13. See FDA, "Pregnant Women."

14. Ibid.

15. See Simpson, "Twin-Twin Transfusion Syndrome," 11.

16. See Asma Khalil, Emily Cooper, Rosemary Townsend, and Basky Thilaganathan, "Evolution of Stage 1 Twin-to-Twin Transfusion Syndrome (TTTS): Systematic Review and Meta-Analysis," *Twin Research and Human Genetics* 19 (2016): 207–16, https://www.cambridge.org/core/journals/twin-research-and-human -genetics/article/evolution-of-stage-1-twintotwin-transfusion-syndrome-ttts -systematic-review-and-metaanalysis/12AD668643BAD32CD802A81B20AF B6FD#fndtn-information, finding a 70 percent double survival rate for TTTS pregnancies treated with expectant management and a 54 percent double survival rate for TTTS pregnancies treated with laser surgery.

17. Computed as the 495 TTTS Stage I (TTTS1) pregnancies studied by Khalil et al., "Evolution of Stage 1 Twin-to-Twin Transfusion Syndrome (TTTS)," plus an additional five TTTS1 pregnancies noted by A. Cristina Rossi and Vincenzo D'Addario in "Survival Outcomes of Twin–Twin transfusion Syndrome Stage I: A Systematic Review of Literature," *American Journal of Obstetrics and Gynecology* 30 (2013): 5–10, table 1, https://www.thieme-connect.com/products/ejournals /abstract/10.1055/s-0032-1322513, and the eleven TTTS1 pregnancies from the Eurofetus Trial reviewed by Marie-Victoire Senat, Jan Deprest, Michel Boulvain, Alain Paupe, Norbert Winer, and Yves Ville, "Endoscopic Laser Surgery versus Serial Amnioreduction for Severe Twin-to-Twin Transfusion Syndrome," *New England Journal of Medicine* 351 (July 2004): 136–44, table 1, https://www.ncbi .nlm.nih.gov/pubmed/15238624. Pregnancies reviewed in more than one article have been deleted from the total.

18. See Senat et al., "Endoscopic Laser Surgery versus Serial Amnioreduction."

19. See Michael W. Bebbington, "Outcomes in a Cohort of Patients with Stage I Twin-to-Twin Transfusion Syndrome," *Ultrasound in Obstetrics and Gynecology* 36 (July 2010): 48–51, Conclusions section, https://obgyn.onlinelibrary.wiley .com/doi/full/10.1002/uog.7612.

Chapter Seven

1. See W. Diehl, A. Diemert, D. Grasso, S. Sehner, K. Wegscheider, and K. Hecher, "Fetoscopic Laser Coagulation in 1020 Pregnancies with Twin-Twin Transfusion

Syndrome Demonstrates Improvement in Double-Twin Survival Rate," *Ultrasound in Obstetrics and Gynecology* 50, no. 6 (December 2017): 728–35, https://obgyn.onlinelibrary.wiley.com/doi/full/10.1002/uog.17520.

2. See E. Gratacós, E. Antolin, L. Lewi, J. M. Martínez, E. Hernandez-Andrade, R. Acosta-Rojas, G. Enríquez, L. Caberom, and J. Deprest, "Monochorionic Twins with Selective Intrauterine Growth Restriction and Intermittent Absent or Reversed End-Diastolic Flow (Type III): Feasibility and Perinatal Outcome of Fetoscopic Placental Laser Coagulation," *Ultrasound in Obstetrics and Gynecology* 31 (2008): 669–75, 673n11, https://obgyn.onlinelibrary.wiley.com/doi/epdf/10.1002/uog.5362.

3. See Gratacós et al., "Monochorionic Twins with Selective Intrauterine Growth Restriction," 674n2.

4. Ibid., 673.

5. See T. Van Mieghem, E. Eixarch, L. Gucciardo, E. Done, I. Gonzales, D. Van Schoubroeck, L. Lewi, E. Gratacós, and J. Deprest, "Outcome Prediction in Monochorionic Diamniotic Twin Pregnancies with Moderately Discordant Amniotic Fluid," *Ultrasound in Obstetrics and Gynecology* 37, no. 1 (January 2011): 15–21, https://obgyn.onlinelibrary.wiley.com/doi/full/10.1002/uog.8802#bib1.

6. See Gratacós et al., "Monochorionic Twins with Selective Intrauterine Growth Restriction," 672n2.

7. Ibid.

8. Julie S. Moldenhauer and Mark P. Johnson, "Diagnosis and Management of Complicated Monochorionic Twins," *Clinical Obstetrics and Gynecology* 58, no. 3 (September 2015): 632–42, https://journals.lww.com/clinicalobgyn/Abstract/2015/09000/Diagnosis_and_Management_of_Complicated.20.aspx.

9. Ibid.

10. Han-jing Chai, Yan-min Luo, Xuan Huang, Yi Zhou, and Qun Fang, "Perinatal Outcome of Monochorionic Diamniotic Twins with Selective Intrauterine Growth Restriction," *Zhonghua Fu Chan Ke Za Zhi* 48, no. 6 (June 2013): 416–20, https://www.ncbi.nlm.nih.gov/m/pubmed/24103119/?i=4&from=/17542039/related (abstract translated into English from the original Chinese).

11. Ibid.

12. See Gratacós et al., "Monochorionic Twins with Selective Intrauterine Growth Restriction," 673n2.

13. See J. M. M. van Klink, H. M. Koopman, J. M. Middeldorp, F. J. Klumper, M. Rijken, D. Oepkes, and E. Lopriore, "Long-Term Neurodevelopmental Outcome after Selective Feticide in Monochorionic Pregnancies," *British Journal of Obstetrics and Gynecology* 122 (2015): 1517–24, assessing neurodevelopmental

outcome in seventy-four long-term survivors. See also van Klink et al., "Randomized Controlled Trials in TTTS," describing long-term follow-up with 216 survivors of laser surgery.

14. See Cardinal Glennon St. Louis Children's Hospital, "Selective Intrauterine Growth Restriction," https://www.ssmhealth.com/cardinal-glennon/fetal-care -institute/twin-abnormalities/selective-intrauterine-growth-restriction. This hospital is Catholic, which could be discerned from the "Cardinal" in its name. Related to fetal therapy, the hospital's website also notes, "Cord occlusion, which involves blocking the umbilical cord of the smaller twin, is not performed at the Cardinal Glennon St. Louis Fetal Care Institute."

15. See Evergreen Health Medical Center, "Fetal Therapy," https://www.evergreen health.com/fetal-therapy.

16. Research from 2014 suggested that TTTS laser surgery could be done after twenty-six weeks of gestation, but I found that most doctors were unfamiliar with studies on expanded timelines for TTTS laser surgery. See David Baud, Rory Windrim, Johannes Keunen, and Greg Ryan, "Fetoscopic Laser Therapy for Twin–Twin Transfusion Syndrome: Beyond Current Gestational Age Limits," *American Journal of Perinatology* 31 (2014): S19–24, https://www.thieme-connect .com/products/ejournals/abstract/10.1055/s-0034-1378143.

17. See FDA, "Humanitarian Device Exemption: Questions and Answers; Draft Guidance for Humanitarian Device Exemption Holders, Institutional Review Boards, Clinical Investigators, and Food and Drug Administration Staff," Docket FDA-2104-D-0223 (March 17, 2014), https://beta.regulations.gov/document /FDA-2014-D-0223-0002. FDA revised this draft guidance in 2018 and asked for public comments on the revisions (see Docket FDA-2014-D-0223-0012, https:// beta.regulations.gov/document/FDA-2014-D-0223-0012); however, the agency never released final guidance on HDEs incorporating the comments received in 2014 and 2018.

18. See Katrina Kimport, "What Happens When Women Planning Abortions View Ultrasounds?," Scholars Strategy Network, July 23, 2015, https://scholars.org /contribution/what-happens-when-women-planning-abortions-view-ultrasounds.

19. See Carol Sanger, "Looking Your Fetus in the Eye: Mandatory Ultrasound and the Politics of Abortion," *Dissent*, November 10, 2009, https://www.dissent magazine.org/online_articles/looking-your-fetus-in-the-eye-mandatory -ultrasound-and-the-politics-of-abortion (citing state examples).

20. Heartbeat Protection Act of 2021, H.R. 705, 117th Congress (2021–22), https:// www.congress.gov/bill/117th-congress/house-bill/705/text.

21. See Kimport, "What Happens When Women Planning Abortions View Ultrasounds?"

22. See Sanger, "Looking Your Fetus in the Eye."

23. See C. Wohlmuth, D. Boudreaux, K. J. Moise Jr., A. Johnson, R. Papanna, M. Bebbington, and H. M. Gardiner, "Cardiac Pathophysiology in Twin-Twin Transfusion Syndrome: New Insights into Its Evolution," *Ultrasound in Obstetrics and Gynecology* 51 (March 2018): 341–48, https://pubmed.ncbi.nlm.nih.gov/28370497/.

24. See Spruijt et al., "Twin-Twin Transfusion Syndrome in the Era of Fetoscopic Laser Surgery," sec. 4, Neonatal Outcome.

25. See Diana Greene Foster and Katrina Kimport, "Who Seeks Abortions at or after 20 Weeks?," *Perspectives on Sexual and Reproductive Health* 45, no. 4 (December 2103): 210–18, https://www.guttmacher.org/journals/psrh/2013/11/who-seeks-abortions-or-after-20-weeks.

26. See Hannah C. Glass, Andrew T. Costarino, Stephen A. Stayer, Claire M. Brett, Franklin Cladis, and Peter J. Davis, "Outcomes for Extremely Premature Infants," *Anesthesia and Analgesia* 120 (June 2015): 1337–51, https://pubmed.ncbi.nlm.nih.gov/25988638/.

27. See Ariana Eunjung Cha, "Tough Questions—and Answers—on 'Late-Term' Abortions, the Law and the Women Who Get Them," *Washington Post*, February 6, 2019, https://www.washingtonpost.com/us-policy/2019/02/06/tough-questions-answers-late-term-abortions-law-women-who-get-them/.

28. Ibid.

29. Ibid.

30. See Guttmacher Institute, "State Bans on Abortion throughout Pregnancy," May 1, 2021, https://www.guttmacher.org/state-policy/explore/state-policies-later-abortions.

31. Ibid.

32. Ibid. See also Jack Healy, "When Can Fetuses Feel Pain? Utah Abortion Law and Doctors Are at Odds," *New York Times*, May 4, 2016, https://www.nytimes.com/2016/05/05/us/utah-abortion-law-fetal-anesthesia.html.

33. See Guttmacher Institute, "State Bans on Abortion throughout Pregnancy."

34. Ibid.

35. Ibid.

36. See Amelia Thomson-DeVeaux, "The Last of the Late-Term Abortion Providers," *American Prospect*, September 20, 2013, https://prospect.org/power/last-late-term-abortion-providers/.

37. The clinic, open when I was pregnant, later closed, and the physician operating it moved to a different location. See Catherine Pearson, "Anti-Abortion Activists Tried to Shut Him Down. One Year Later, His Clinic Is Thriving," *Huffington Post*, October 30, 2018, https://www.huffpost.com/entry/anti-abortion-activists-tried-to-shut-him-down-one-year-later-his-clinic-is-thriving_n_5bc4cce8e4b01a01d68d508e.

38. See Brian Palmer, "Mommy, Where Do Pictures of Aborted Babies Come From?," *Slate*, October 26, 2010, https://slate.com/news-and-politics/2010/10/where-do-anti-abortion-protesters-get-those-grisly-photos.html.

39. See, e.g., Joan Finn-McCracken, "I Helped Women Get Abortions for 28 Years—Through Protests and Shifting Rules," *Washington Post*, May 25, 2018, https://www.washingtonpost.com/outlook/i-helped-women-get-abortions-for-28-years--through-protests-and-shifting-rules/2018/05/25/4f680826-5eb8-11e8-a4a4-c070ef53f315_story.html, describing how abortion protesters may seek abortions for themselves or for their pregnant daughters.

40. Written comments of Dr. Kathryn Marko, February 28, 2021.

41. See Glass et al., "Outcomes for Extremely Premature Infants."

42. See Diane Christopher, Barrett K. Robinson, and Alan M. Peaceman, "An Evidence-Based Approach to Determining Route of Delivery for Twin Gestations," *Review of Obstetrics and Gynecology* 4, no. 3–4 (2011): 109–16, https://www.ncbi.nlm.nih.gov/pmc/articles/PMC3252881/.

43. See Glass et al., "Outcomes for Extremely Premature Infants," Survival and Morbidity section.

44. Ibid.

45. See Sara Novak, "How Long Will My Premature Baby Stay in the NICU?," What to Expect, February 3, 2020, https://www.whattoexpect.com/first-year/preemie-categorization/.

46. See Glass et al., "Outcomes for Extremely Premature Infants," fig. 4.

47. See Emile Papiernik et al., "Differences in Outcome between Twins and Singletons Born Very Preterm: Results from a Population-based European Cohort," *Human Reproduction* 25, no. 4 (April 2010): 1035–43, https://www.ncbi.nlm.nih.gov/pubmed/20118116.

48. See Morrison, "Twin Gestation and Premature Birth."

49. Ibid.

50. Ibid.

51. See Glass et al., "Outcomes for Extremely Premature Infants."

52. See Kevin Perez, "Developmental Risks Remain High among Premature Babies

despite Improved Survival Rates, French Study Shows," *Cerebral Palsy News Today*, August 30, 2017, https://cerebralpalsynewstoday.com/2017/08/30/cerebral -palsy-decreases-among-premature-babies-but-risk-of-developmental-delay -remains-high-france-study-shows/.

53. See Glass et al., "Outcomes for Extremely Premature Infants."

54. See Mikko Hirvonen, Ritta Ojala, Päivi Korhonen, Paula Haataja, Kai Eriksson, Mika Gissler, Tiina Luukkaala, and Outi Tammela, "Cerebral Palsy among Children Born Moderately and Late Preterm," *Pediatrics* 134, no. 6 (December 2014): 1584–93, https://pediatrics.aappublications.org/content/134/6/e1584.

55. See Dag Moster, Allen J. Wilcox, Stein Emil Vollset, Trond Markestad, and Rolv Terje Lie, "Cerebral Palsy among Term and Post-Term Births," *JAMA* 304, no. 9 (September 2010), 976–82, https://www.ncbi.nlm.nih.gov/pmc/articles /PMC3711561/.

56. See Morrison, "Twin Gestation and Premature Birth."

Chapter Eight

1. See Zehra Nihal Dolgun, Cihan Inan, Ahmet Salih Altintas, Sabri Berkem Okten, and Niyazi Cenk Sayin, "Preterm Birth in Twin Pregnancies: Clinical Outcomes and Predictive Parameters," *Pakistani Journal of Medical Science* 32, no. 4 (July–August 2016): 922–26, 925, https://www.ncbi.nlm.nih.gov/pmc /articles/PMC5017103/.

2. See Caroline Crowther and Shanshan Han, "Hospitalisation and Bed Rest for Multiple Pregnancy," Cochrane Database of Systematic Reviews, July 7, 2010, https://pubmed.ncbi.nlm.nih.gov/11279677/.

3. See Anthony C. Sciscione, "Maternal Activity Restriction and the Prevention of Preterm Birth," *American Journal of Obstetrics and Gynecology* 202, no. 3 (March 2010): 232.e1–5, https://pubmed.ncbi.nlm.nih.gov/19766979/.

4. See Maritza M. Fujita, Maria L. Brizot, Adolfo W. Liao, Tatiana Bernáth, Luciana Cury, Jorge D. Banduki Neto, and Marcelo Zugaib, "Reference Range for Cervical Length in Twin Pregnancies," *Acta Obstetricia et Gynecologica Scandinavica* 81, no. 9 (September 2002): 856–59, https://obgyn.onlinelibrary.wiley .com/doi/full/10.1034/j.1600-0412.2002.810910.x.

5. See Ingrid Bergelin and Lil Valentin, "Cervical Changes in Twin Pregnancies Observed by Transvaginal Ultrasound during the Latter Half of Pregnancy: A Longitudinal, Observational Study," *Ultrasound in Obstetrics and Gynecology* 21, no. 6 (June 2003): 556–63, https://obgyn.onlinelibrary.wiley.com/doi /full/10.1002/uog.150.

6. See Zehra Nihal Dolgun, Cihan Inan, Ahmet Salih Altintas, Sabri Berkem Okten, and Niyazi Cenk Sayin, "Preterm Birth in Twin Pregnancies: Clinical Outcomes and Predictive Parameters," *Pakistani Journal of Medical Science* 32, no. 4 (July–August 2016): 922–26, 925, https://www.ncbi.nlm.nih.gov/pmc/articles/PMC5017103/.

7. See J. Dor, J. Shalev, S. Mashiach, J. Blankstein, and D. M. Serr, "Elective Cervical Suture of Twin Pregnancies Diagnosed Ultrasonically in the First Trimester Following Induced Ovulation," *Gynecolic and Obstetric Investigation* 13, no. 1 (1982): 55–60, https://pubmed.ncbi.nlm.nih.gov/7056503/.

8. See American College of Obstetricians and Gynecologists (ACOG), "Periviable Birth," *Obstetric Care Consensus* 130, no. 6 (October 2017): e187–99, https://www.acog.org/clinical/clinical-guidance/obstetric-care-consensus/articles/2017/10/periviable-birth. This guidance document was updated with new information in 2019.

9. Ibid.

10. See Marcelo Santucci Franca, Tatiana E. N. K. Hamamoto, and Antônio Fernandes Moron, "Preterm Birth in Twins," *Multiple Pregnancy—New Challenges* (2018), secs. 3.3 and 3.5, https://www.intechopen.com/books/multiple-pregnancy-new-challenges/preterm-birth-in-twins, on beta-antagonists.

11. See TTTS Foundation, "Good Habits and Ways to Help Yourself: Cervical Assessment, Nutritional Therapy, and Bedrest," http://www.tttsfoundation.org/help_during_pregnancy/summary.php.

12. See also J. E. De Lia, R. S. Kuhlmann, and M. G. Emery, "Maternal Metabolic Abnormalities in Twin-to-Twin Transfusion Syndrome at Mid-Pregnancy," *Twin Research*, 3, no. 2 (June 2000): 113–17, https://pubmed.ncbi.nlm.nih.gov/10918625, noting maternal hypoproteinemia of women with TTTS pregnancies but providing no evidence about the utility of drinking mass quantities of protein.

13. I do not know what my spouse's excuse was for not realizing the precise location of the new house. In revisionist history, he now claims that he knew it was in DC all along.

14. See Alexandra Sacks, "Reframing 'Mommy Brain,'" *New York Times*, May 11, 2018, https://www.nytimes.com/2018/05/11/well/family/reframing-mommy-brain.html.

15. See Pam Belluck, "Pregnancy Changes the Brain in Ways That May Help Mothering," *New York Times*, December 19, 2016, https://www.nytimes.com/2016/12/19/health/pregnancy-brain-change.html.

16. See Anna Ziomkiewicz, Szymon Wichary, and Grazyna Jasienska, "Cognitive Costs of Reproduction: Life-History Trade-Offs Explain Cognitive Decline during Pregnancy in Women," *Biological Reviews* 94, no. 3 (June 2019): 1105–15, https://pubmed.ncbi.nlm.nih.gov/30588733/.

17. See Ann-Marie G. Lange, Claudia Barth, Tobias Kaufmann, Melis Anatürk, Sana Suri, Klaus P. Ebmeier, and Lars T. Westlye, "The Maternal Brain: Region-Specific Patterns of Brain Aging Are Traceable Decades after Childbirth," *Human Brain Mapping* 41, no. 16 (2020): 4718–29, 4719, https://onlinelibrary.wiley.com/doi/10.1002/hbm.25152.

18. See Belluck, "Pregnancy Changes the Brain."

19. See Sachs, "Reframing 'Mommy Brain.'"

20. See Belluck, "Pregnancy Changes the Brain."

21. See Lange et al., "The Maternal Brain," 4726.

22. Studies of new fathers found no similar effect. See Belluck, "Pregnancy Changes the Brain."

23. See Cindy K. Barha and Liisa A. M. Galea, "The Maternal 'Baby Brain' Revisited," *Nature Neuroscience* 20 (2017): 134–35, https://www.nature.com/articles/nn.4473.

24. See Lange et al., "The Maternal Brain," 4726.

25. Ibid., 4722.

26. See Alice Callahan, "Should You Give Birth at a Birth Center?," *New York Times*, September 25, 2018, https://www.nytimes.com/2018/09/25/well/family/should-you-give-birth-at-a-birth-center.html.

27. See March of Dimes, "Levels of Medical Care for Your Newborn," March 2015, https://www.marchofdimes.org/baby/levels-of-medical-care-for-your-newborn.aspx. In researching for this book, I learned that maternal care facilities are also rated according to their level of specialty and skill. No one ever mentioned these labor and delivery ward ratings to me when I was pregnant. All focus was on the level of care the twins would receive. The care I would receive simply was not a known factor for my decision-making.

28. See CHOP, "Survival Rates in High Level NICUs Better than Previously Noted," CHOP News, July 23, 2012, https://www.chop.edu/news/survival-rates-high-level-nicus-better-previously-noted.

29. Ibid.

30. See Stephan N. Wall, Anne C. C. Lee, Susan Niermeyer, Mike English, William J. Keenan, Wally Carlo, Zulfiqar A. Bhutta, Abhay Bang, Indira Narayanan, Iwan Ariawan, and Joy E. Lawn, "Neonatal Resuscitation in Low-Resource

Settings: What, Who, and How to Overcome Challenges to Scale Up?," *International Journal of Gynaecology and Obstetrics* 107, suppl. 1 (October 2009): S47–64, https://www.ncbi.nlm.nih.gov/pmc/articles/PMC2875104/.

31. See ACOG, "Periviable Birth," e188.

32. Ibid.

33. See Clarissa Gutierrez Carvalho, "Ventilator-Induced Lung Injury in Preterm Infants," *Revista brasileira de terapia intensiva* 25, no. 4 (October–December 2013): 319–26, 320, https://www.ncbi.nlm.nih.gov/pmc/articles/PMC4031878/.

34. See ACOG, "Periviable Birth," e189.

35. Ibid.

36. See William L. Meadow and John D. Lantos, "Ethics, Data, and Policy in Newborn Intensive Care," in *Avery's Diseases of the Newborn*, 9th ed., edited by Christine A. Gleason and Sandra E. Juul, 20–24, 23 (Philadelphia: Elsevier, 2012), http://seciss.facmed.unam.mx/wp-content/uploads/2021/01/Averys-Diseases-of -the-Newborn-10th-Edition-2018-1.pdf.

37. One set of authors has proposed a new framework for neonatal resuscitation not based on gestational age but rather prognosticated outcome from mechanical ventilation. If a poor outcome is 50 to 90 percent likely, then the parents' wishes related to resuscitation should be followed. See Lynn Gillam, Dominic Wilkinson, Vicki Xafis, and David Isaacs, "Decision-Making at the Borderline of Viability: Who Should Decide and on What Basis?," *Journal of Paediatrics and Child Health* 53, no. 2 (February 2017): 105–11, 106, table 2, https://pubmed.ncbi .nlm.nih.gov/28194892/.

38. See Myra H. Wyckoff, Khalid Aziz, Marilyn B. Escobedo, Vishal S. Kapadia, John Kattwinkel, Jeffrey M. Perlman, Wendy M. Simon, Gary M. Weiner, and Jeanette G. Zaichkin, "Neonatal Resuscitation: 2015 American Heart Association Guidelines Update for Cardiopulmonary Resuscitation and Emergency Cardiovascular Care," *Pediatrics* 136, suppl. 2 (2015): S195–218, S205, https:// pediatrics.aappublications.org/content/136/Supplement_2/S196#sec-35.

39. Ibid., S204.

40. See Meadow and Lantos, "Ethics, Data, and Policy in Newborn Intensive Care," 23.

41. See Matthew A. Rysavy et al., "Between-Hospital Variation in Treatment and Outcomes in Extremely Preterm Infants," *New England Journal of Medicine* 372, no. 19 (May 7, 2015): 1801–11, https://www.ncbi.nlm.nih.gov/pmc/articles /PMC4465092/, examining resuscitation policies at twenty-four US hospitals for babies born before twenty-seven weeks of gestation and finding wide, unexplained differences in the provision of resuscitation.

42. See Gillam et al., "Decision-Making at the Borderline of Viability," 108.

43. Ibid., 105.

44. Miller v. HCA, Inc., 118 S.W.3rd 758 (Texas 2003), https://search.txcourts.gov
    /SearchMedia.aspx?MediaVersionID=de3efae4-d550-4799-a5a5-519d93bc778d
    &coa=cossup&DT=OPINION&MediaID=079e64d2-eec7-4bea-8b3d
    -ed47b9cf083c.

45. See George J. Annas, "Extremely Preterm Birth and Parental Authority to Refuse
    Treatment—The Case of Sidney Miller," *New England Journal of Medicine* 351
    (November 2004): 2118–23, 2118, https://www.nejm.org/doi/full/10.1056
    /nejmlim041201.

46. See Brian M. Cummings, Mark R. Mercurio, and John J. Paris, "A Review of Ap-
    proaches for Resolving Disputes between Physicians and Families on End-of-Life
    Care for Newborns," *Journal of Perinatology* 40 (May 2020): 1441–45, https://
    www.nature.com/articles/s41372-020-0675-4.

47. See Louise Melling, "Before You Go to a Catholic Hospital, Read This," ACLU
    blog, December 19, 2013, https://www.aclu.org/blog/religious-liberty/using
    -religion-discriminate/you-go-catholic-hospital-read.

48. United States Conference of Catholic Bishops (USCCB), *Ethical and Religious
    Directives for Catholic Health Care Services*, 6th ed. (2016), 21, nos. 56 and 57,
    https://www.usccb.org/about/doctrine/ethical-and-religious-directives
    /upload/ethical-religious-directives-catholic-health-service-sixth-edition
    -2016-06.pdf.

49. James McTavish, "Decision Making in Neonatal End-of-Life Scenarios in Low-
    Income Settings," *Linacre Quarterly* 84, no. 3 (May 2017): 232–42, 236, https://
    www.tandfonline.com/doi/abs/10.1080/00243639.2017.1300759.

50. See Rebecca Cooper, "Delivery Room Resuscitation of the High-Risk Infant:
    A Conflict of Rights," *Catholic Lawyer* 33, no. 4 (1990): 325–60, 333, https://
    scholarship.law.stjohns.edu/tcl/vol33/iss4/5/.

51. See McTavish, "Decision Making in Neonatal End-of-Life Scenarios in Low-
    Income Setting."

52. See ACLU and MergerWatch, "The Growth of Catholic Hospitals and Health
    Care: 2016 Update to the Miscarriage of Medicine Report," 2016, http://static1
    .1.sqspcdn.com/static/f/816571/27061007/1465224862580/MW_Update-2016
    -MiscarrOfMedicine-report.pdf.

53. Ibid.

54. Ibid., noting the number of acute care facilities dropped by six percent from 2001
    to 2016. See also Frédéric Michas, "Number of All Hospitals in the U.S. from
    1975 to 2018," *Statista*, December 1, 2020, https://www.statista.com/statistics

/185843/number-of-all-hospitals-in-the-us-since-2001/, demonstrating the decrease in registered and unregistered hospitals from 2001 to 2020.

55. See Robin Warshaw, "Health Disparities Affect Millions in Rural U.S. Communities," AAMCNews, October 31, 2017, https://www.aamc.org/news-insights/health-disparities-affect-millions-rural-us-communities, citing a study published in *Health Affairs* that found "45 percent of all rural US counties, where nearly two million women of reproductive age lived in 2004, had no hospital-based obstetric services in the period 2004–14. Another 9 percent of counties, where more than 650,000 reproductive-age women lived in 2004, lost obstetric services during the study period, leaving more than half of all rural US counties without obstetric services."

56. See Della A. Campbell, Marian F. Lake, Michele Falk, and Jeffrey R. Bacstrand, "A Randomized Control Trial of Continuous Support in Labor by a Lay Doula," *Journal of Obstetric, Gynecologic, and Neonatal Nursing* 35, no. 4 (July–August 2006): 456–64, https://pubmed.ncbi.nlm.nih.gov/16881989/.

57. See Kenneth J. Gruber, Susan H. Cupito, and Christina F. Dobson, "Impact of Doulas on Healthy Birth Outcomes," *Journal of Perinatal Education* 22, no. 1 (Winter 2013): 49–58, https://pubmed.ncbi.nlm.nih.gov/24381478/.

58. See Campbell et al., "A Randomized Control Trial of Continuous Support in Labor by a Lay Doula," Results section.

59. See Gruber et al., "Impact of Doulas on Healthy Birth Outcomes," 50.

60. DONA International, "Benefits of a Doula," https://www.dona.org/what-is-a-doula/benefits-of-a-doula/.

61. See, for instance, Claire Ridgway, "Mary I's Will," Tudor Society, https://www.tudorsociety.com/mary-is-will/ (on the queen's last will and testament). See also Claire Ridgway, "Childbirth in Medieval and Tudor Times by Sarah Bryson," Tudor Society, https://www.tudorsociety.com/childbirth-in-medieval-and-tudor-times-by-sarah-bryson/, and Victoria and Albert Museum, "Renaissance Childbirth" (2016), http://www.vam.ac.uk/content/articles/r/renaissance-childbirth/.

62. See Geoffrey Chamberlain, "British Maternal Mortality in the 19th and Early 20th Centuries," *Journal of the Royal Society of Medicine* 99, no. 11 (November 2006): 559–63, 559, https://www.ncbi.nlm.nih.gov/pmc/articles/PMC1633559/.

63. See Martin and Montagne, "U.S. Has the Worst Rate of Maternal Deaths in the Developed World."

64. See Natalie Rahhal, "Half of US States Refuse to Honor Pregnant Women's Living Wills—and 12 Keep Them Alive as 'Fetal Containers' if They Die before Childbirth, Study Finds," *Daily Mail*, April 23, 2019, https://www.dailymail.co

.uk/health/article-6950743/Half-states-refuse-honor-pregnant-womens-living
-wills.html.

65. See Elizabeth Villarreal, "Pregnancy and Living Wills: A Behavioral Economic
Analysis," *Yale Law Journal Forum* 128 (April 2019): 1052–76, 1052, https://www
.yalelawjournal.org/pdf/Villarreal_huru3n6p.pdf.

66. See Rahhal, "Half of US States Refuse to Honor Pregnant Women's Living
Wills."

67. See Villarreal, "Pregnancy and Living Wills," 1053, footnote 7 and table 1.

68. See Rahhal, "Half of US States Refuse to Honor Pregnant Women's Living
Wills," map.

69. Alex Farr, Frank A. Chervenak, Laurence B. McCullough, Rebecca N. Baergen,
and Amos Grünebaum, "Human Placentophagy: A Review," *American Journal
of Obstetrics and Gynecology* 218, no. 4 (April 2018): 401.e1–11, https://www.ajog
.org/article/S0002-9378(17)30963-8/fulltext. See also Mark B. Kristal, Jean M.
DiPirro, and Alexis C. Thompson, "Placentophagia in Humans and Nonhuman
Mammals: Causes and Consequences," *Ecology of Food and Nutrition* 51, no. 3
May 2012): 177–97, https://www.acsu.buffalo.edu/~kristal/placentophagia%20
review.pdf.

70. See Genevieve L. Buser, Sayonara Mató, Alexia Y. Zhang, Ben J. Metcalf, Bernard
Beall, and Ann R. Thomas, "Notes from the Field: Late-Onset Infant Group B
Streptococcus Infection Associated with Maternal Consumption of Capsules
Containing Dehydrated Placenta—Oregon, 2016," *Morbidity and Mortality
Weekly Report* 66, no. 25 (June 2017): 677–78, http://dx.doi.org/10.15585/mmwr
.mm6625a4.

Chapter Nine

1. Enrico Lopriore, Liesbeth Lewi, and Asma Khalil, "Monochorionic Twins: A
Delicate Balance," *Journal of Clinical Medicine* 8, no. 10 (October 2019): 1711–13,
1712, https://www.ncbi.nlm.nih.gov/pmc/articles/PMC6832893/.

2. Ibid.

3. See Bonnie Kristian, "The Double Disadvantage of Twin Pregnancies in America," *The Week*, February 25, 2019, https://theweek.com/articles/824777/double
-disadvantage-twin-pregnancies-america.

4. See Jon F. R. Barrett et al., "A Randomized Trial of Planned Cesarean or Vaginal
Delivery for Twin Pregnancy," *New England Journal of Medicine* 369 (October
2013): 1295–1305, https://www.nejm.org/doi/full/10.1056/nejmoa1214939.

5. See Sau Lan Mok and Tsz Kin Lo, "Long Term Outcome of Second Twins Born

to Mothers Who Attempted Vaginal Delivery: A Retrospective Study," *European Journal of Obstetrics and Gynecology and Reproductive Biology* 254 (November 2020): 1–5, https://doi.org/10.1016/j.ejogrb.2020.08.049.

6. See Amir Aviram, Hayley Lipworth, Elizabeth V. Asztalos, Elad Mei-Dan, Nir Melamed, Xingshan Cao, Arthur Zaltz, Lone Hvidman, and Jon F. R. Barrett, "Delivery of Monochorionic Twins: Lessons Learned from the Twin Birth Study," *American Journal of Obstetrics and Gynecology* 223 (June 2020): 916.e1–9, https://pubmed.ncbi.nlm.nih.gov/32592694/.

7. See Simone M. T. A. Goossens, Sabine Ensing, Mark A. H. B. M. van der Hoeven, Frans J. M. E. Roumen, Jan G. Nijhuis, and Ben W. Mol, "Comparison of Planned Caesarean Delivery and Planned Vaginal Delivery in Women with a Twin Pregnancy: A Nationwide Cohort Study," *European Journal of Obstetrics and Reproductive Gynecology* 221 (February 2018): 97–104, https://doi.org/10.1016/j.ejogrb.2017.12.018.

8. Ibid.

9. Ibid.

10. See Christopher et al., "An Evidence-Based Approach to Determining Route of Delivery for Twin Gestations," table 1.

11. See Zarko Alfirevic, Stefan J. Milan, and Stefania Livio, "Caesarean Section versus Vaginal Delivery for Preterm Birth in Singletons," Cochrane Database of Systematic Reviews 6, no. 6, CD000078 (June 2012); update in Cochrane Database of Systematic Reviews 9 CD000078 (September 2013), http://www.ncbi.nlm.nih.gov/pubmed/22696314.

12. See Mok and Lo, "Long Term Outcome of Second Twins."

13. See Christopher et al., "An Evidence-Based Approach to Determining Route of Delivery for Twin Gestations," 110, fig. 1, notes 5 and 9.

14. Ibid., 110, fig. 1. My ob/gyn insists that I note the concern for sIUGR babies and vaginal delivery is more the inability to "tolerate labor." A growth restricted baby often has a bigger head than its abdominal circumference, leading to a higher risk of head entrapment in the mother's cervix while the baby is being born. This is more common in larger babies, weighing 1500–2500 grams, or for twins where the first presenting twin is much smaller than the other twin. Such a situation was the opposite of mine, though, as both my twins were very small, and the larger twin was the one positioned to be born first. Written comments of Dr. Kathryn Marko, Feb. 28, 2021, in author's and publisher's possession.

15. See Christopher et al., "An Evidence-Based Approach to Determining Route of Delivery for Twin Gestations," 112.

16. Dinoprostone would be used, not misoprostol, the ripening agent used in Europe.

17. See Mayo Clinic, "Labor Induction," https://www.mayoclinic.org/tests -procedures/labor-induction/about/pac-20385141.

18. See National Institutes of Health, "Induced Labor at 39 Weeks May Reduce Likelihood of C-section, NIH Study Suggests," August 8, 2018, https://www.nih .gov/news-events/news-releases/induced-labor-39-weeks-may-reduce-likelihood -c-section-nih-study-suggests.

19. See Maria Jonsson, "Induction of Twin Pregnancy and the Risk of Caesarean Delivery: A Cohort Study," *BMC Pregnancy Childbirth* 15, no. 1 (2015): 136–42, https://doi.org/10.1186/s12884-015-0566-4.

20. Ibid.

21. See Armin S. Razavi, Stephen T. Chasen, Fiona Chambers, and Robin B. Kalish, "Maternal Morbidity Associated with Labor Induction in Twin Gestations," *American Journal of Obstetrics and Gynecology*, suppl. (January 2017): S427, https://www.ajog.org/article/S0002-9378(16)31446-6/pdf.

22. See Judith A. Lothian, "Saying 'No' to Induction," *Journal of Perinatal Education* 15, no. 2 (Spring 2006): 43–45, https://www.ncbi.nlm.nih.gov/pmc/articles /PMC1595289/.

23. See ACOG, "Medications for Pain Relief During Labor and Delivery: Frequently Asked Questions," April 2019, https://www.acog.org/womens-health/faqs /medications-for-pain-relief-during-labor-and-delivery.

24. See Kristian, "The Double Disadvantage of Twin Pregnancies in America."

25. See Rebecca Dekker, "Evidence on: Eating and Drinking during Labor," Evidence Based Birth, February 2017, https://evidencebasedbirth.com/evidence-eating -drinking-labor/.

26. Ibid., citing T. M. Cook, N. Woodall, and C. Frerk, "Major Complications of Airway Management in the UK: Results of the Fourth National Audit Project of the Royal College of Anaesthetists and the Difficult Airway Society; Part 1: Anaesthesia," *British Journal of Anaesthesia* 106 (May 2011): 617–31, https:// pubmed.ncbi.nlm.nih.gov/21447488/.

27. See Beverley Chalmers, "Maternity Care in the Former Soviet Union," *British Journal of Obstetrics and Gynaecology* 112, no. 4 (April 2005): 495–99, 496, https:// obgyn.onlinelibrary.wiley.com/doi/pdf/10.1111/j.1471-0528.2005.00626.x.

28. Jenny McCarthy, *Belly Laughs: The Naked Truth about Pregnancy and Childbirth* (Boston: Da Capo, 2005).

29. See Cara Terreri, "Will I Really Poop During Birth," Top 10 Childbirth Fears, November 6, 2015, https://www.lamaze.org/Giving-Birth-with-Confidence

/GBWC-Post/top-10-childbirth-fears-a-series-will-i-really-poop-during-birth. See also Colleen de Bellefonds, "What Really Happens during Labor," What to Expect, March 21, 2019, https://www.whattoexpect.com/pregnancy/photo-gallery /what-really-happens-during-labor.aspx.

30. See Maame Yaa A. B. Yiadom, "What Are the Mortality Rates for Postpartum Hemorrhage (PPH)?," Medscape.com, January 2, 2018, https://www.medscape .com/answers/796785-122141/what-are-the-mortality-rates-for-postpartum -hemorrhage-pph.

31. Ibid.

32. See Claire Ngozo, "Malawi: Putting Knowledge into Practice in Childbirth," Inter Press Service News Agency, March 31, 2011, http://www.ipsnews.net/2011 /03/malawi-putting-knowledge-into-practice-in-childbirth/.

33. See Summer Sherburne Hawkins, "Maternal Mortality Is Worse in Washington, D.C. than Syria. Abortion Access Is One Reason Why," Think, NBCNews .com, February 18, 2020, https://www.nbcnews.com/think/opinion/maternal -mortality-worse-washington-d-c-syria-abortion-access-one-ncna1136446.

34. See United Nations, Department of Economic and Social Affairs, Statistics Division, Series: Maternal Mortality Ratio SH_STA_MORT, SDG (Sustainable Development Goals) Indicators, https://unstats.un.org/sdgs/indicators/database/ (select Goal 3, Target 3.1, and Indicator 3.1.1, Maternal Mortality Ratio).

35. See Dan L. Ellsbury, Reese H. Clark, Robert Ursprung, Darren L. Handler, Elizabeth D. Dodd, and Alan R. Spitzer, "A Multifaceted Approach to Improving Outcomes in the NICU: The Pediatrix 100 000 Babies Campaign," *Pediatrics* 137, no. 4 (April 2016): e20150389, https://pediatrics.aappublications.org/content /137/4/e20150389.

36. See Erik A. Jensen and Scott A. Lorch, "Effects of a Birth Hospital's Neonatal Intensive Care Unit Level and Annual Volume of Very Low-Birth-Weight Infant Deliveries on Morbidity and Mortality," *JAMA Pediatrics* 169 (August 2015): e151906, https://jamanetwork.com/journals/jamapediatrics/fullarticle/2399513.

37. Ibid., Discussion section.

38. Ibid.

39. See Ellsbury et al., "A Multifaceted Approach to Improving Outcomes in the NICU," Model Development section.

40. See Genevieve Allen and Naomi Laventhal, "Should Long-Term Consequences of NICU Care Be Discussed in Terms of Prognostic Uncertainty or Possible Harm?," *AMA Journal of Ethics* 19, no. 8 (2017): 743–52, https://journalofethics .ama-assn.org/article/should-long-term-consequences-nicu-care-be-discussed -terms-prognostic-uncertainty-or-possible-harm/2017-08.

41. See Ellsbury et al., "A Multifaceted Approach to Improving Outcomes in the NICU," table 2.

42. See Ravi Mangal Patel, Matthew A. Rysavy, Edward F. Bell, and Jon E. Tyson, "Survival of Infants Born at Periviable Gestational Ages," *Clinics in Perinatology* 44, no. 2 (2017): 287–303, fig. 5, https://www.ncbi.nlm.nih.gov/pmc/articles /PMC5424630/.

43. See Ellsbury et al., "A Multifaceted Approach to Improving Outcomes in the NICU," Discussion section.

Chapter Ten

1. See Cheryl Bird, "Should Twins and Multiples Co-Bed in the NICU?," Verywell Family, November 26, 2020, https://www.verywellfamily.com/should-twins -sleep-together-in-the-nicu-2748591.

2. See Melissa Cox, "When Can My Baby Go Home? Milestones NICU Babies Need to Meet before Being Discharged," University of Louisville Physicians blog, December 11, 2019, https://uoflphysicians.com/blog/2019/12/11/when-can-my -baby-go-home-milestones-nicu-babies-need-to-meet-before-being-discharged/.

3. See, e.g., Maryland Department of Health and Mental Hygiene, "Children and Youth with Special Health Care Needs Accessible Resource Locator," http:// specialneeds.health.maryland.gov/SimpleNav.aspx?keywordId=153, listing the home-based care nursing agencies in Maryland.

4. District of Columbia Department of Health, "Home Health Aide Regulations, Notice of Final Rulemaking," September 9, 2017, sec. 9305, Certification by Examination, https://dchealth.dc.gov/sites/default/files/dc/sites/doh/publication /attachments/Home%20Health%20Aide%20Regulations%20-%20Final%209 -29-2017_0.pdf.

5. Ibid., sec. 9307, Renewal of Certification.

6. See Home Health Aide Guide, Maryland HHA Requirements, https://www .homehealthaideguide.com/hha-training/states/maryland-hha/.

7. See "D.C. Ranks Worst Place in the Nation for Nurses," May 5, 2017, DC Refined, http://dcrefined.com/city-living/dc-ranks-worst-place-in-the-nation -for-nurses.

8. See Dennis Hevesi, "Katie Beckett, Who Inspired Health Reform, Dies at 34," *New York Times*, May 22, 2012, https://www.nytimes.com/2012/05/23/us/katie -beckett-who-inspired-health-reform-dies-at-34.html.

9. See Department of Health Care Finance, District of Columbia, "Tax Equity and Fiscal Responsibility Act (TEFRA) / Katie Beckett," https://dhcf.dc.gov/service /tax-equity-and-fiscal-responsibility-act-tefrakatie-beckett.

10. See MaryBeth Musumeci and Priya Chidambaram, "A Look at Eligibility, Services, and Spending," Kaiser Family Foundation Issue Brief, June 2019, 2, http://files.kff.org/attachment/Medicaid%E2%80%99s-Role-for-Children-with-Special-Health-Care-Needs-A-Look-at-Eligibility,-Services-and-Spending.

11. See Carolyn C. Foster, Rishi K. Agarwal, and Matthew M. Davis, "Home Health Care for Children with Medical Complexity: Workforce Gaps, Policy, and Future Directions," *Health Affairs* 38, no. 6 (June 2019): 987–93, 988, https://www.healthaffairs.org/doi/full/10.1377/hlthaff.2018.05531.

12. See Musumeci and Chidambaram, "Medicaid's Role for Children with Special Health Care Needs," 5.

13. See Tara Anne Pleat, "Katie Beckett Waiver Brings Home Care to Kids with Serious Disabilities," Special Needs Alliance, https://www.specialneedsalliance.org/blog/katie-beckett-waiver-brings-home-care-to-kids-with-serious-disabilities/.

14. See Musumeci and Chidambaram, "Medicaid's Role for Children with Special Health Care Needs," 3.

15. See Tricia Brooks and Allexa Gardner, "Snapshot of Children with Medicaid by Race and Ethnicity, 2018," Georgetown University Health Policy Institute Center for Children and Families, July 2020, https://ccf.georgetown.edu/wp-content/uploads/2020/07/Snapshot-Medicaid-kids-race-ethnicity-v4.pdf.

16. See Chambliss Law, "HHS Establishes Deadline for Use of Provider Relief Fund Distributions," Legal Update, July 31, 2020, https://www.chamblisslaw.com/hhs-establishes-deadline-for-use-of-provider-relief-fund-distributions/.

17. A valid criticism of international assistance is that a lactation consultant could be a twenty-year-old, nulliparous woman. Another book will have to examine those issues.

18. A "Karen" is a 2020s meme of an officious white woman who, secure in her privilege, sticks her nose exactly where it never belonged, often endangering the lives of people of color. See Ashitha Nagesh, "What Exactly Is a 'Karen' and Where Did the Meme Come From?," BBC News, July 30, 2020, https://www.bbc.com/news/world-53588201.

19. See American Academy of Pediatrics, *Federal Support for Breastfeeding*, https://ucsdcommunityhealth.org/wp-content/uploads/2016/04/AAP-Federal-Support-for-Breastfeeding-Summary-2013.pdf, referencing sections 2713 and 4207, respectively, of the Patient Protection and Affordable Care Act of 2010, also known as Obamacare.

20. See Human Milk Banking Association of North America, "Find a Milk Bank," https://www.hmbana.org/find-a-milk-bank/.

21. See FDA, "Use of Donor Human Milk," Science and Research Special Topics, March 22, 2018, https://www.fda.gov/science-research/pediatrics/use-donor -human-milk.

Chapter Eleven

1. See Bamberg and Hecher, "Update on Twin-to-Twin Transfusion Syndrome," 58.
2. See Saulo Molina Giraldo, Ramesh Papanna, K. J. Moise, and Anthony Johnson, "Management of Stage I Twin-to-Twin Transfusion Syndrome: An International Survey," *Ultrasound in Obstetrics and Gynecology* 36, no. 1 (July 2010): 42–47, https://www.researchgate.net/publication/41149501_Management_of_Stage_I _twin-to-twin_transfusion_syndrome_an_international_survey.
3. See Khalil et al., "Evolution of Stage 1 Twin-to-Twin Transfusion Syndrome (TTTS)," table 1, citing eight studies of 147 twin pregnancies complicated by Quintero Stage 1 TTTS and managed by amnioreduction.
4. See Liesbeth Lewi, "Monochorionic Diamniotic Twins: What Do I Tell the Pro-spective Parents?," *Prenatal Diagnosis* 40, no. 7 (June 2020): 766–75, sec. 7.2, In-trafetal or Cord Coagulation, https://obgyn.onlinelibrary.wiley.com/doi/10.1002 /pd.5705.
5. See Mauro Parra-Cordero, Mar Bennesar, José Martínez, Elisenda Eixarch, Ximena Torres, and Eduard Gratacós, "Cord Occlusion in Monochorionic Twins with Early Selective Intrauterine Growth Restriction and Abnormal Umbilical Artery Doppler: A Consecutive Series of 90 Cases," *Fetal Diagnosis and Therapy* 39 (2016): 186–91, https://pubmed.ncbi.nlm.nih.gov/26344150/. However, a 2020 review of relatively few TTTS pregnancies treated with cord occlusion found 50 percent of these resulted in preterm birth before thirty-two weeks of the surviv-ing twin. See Daniela Murgano et al., "Outcome of Twin-to-Twin Transfusion Syndrome in Monochorionic Monoamniotic Twin Pregnancy: Systematic Review and Meta-Analysis," *Ultrasound in Obstetrics and Gynecology* 55, no. 3 (March 2020): 310–17, https://pubmed.ncbi.nlm.nih.gov/31595578/.
6. See Lewi, "Monochorionic Diamniotic Twins."
7. See Marie-Victoire Senat, Jan Deprest, Michel Boulvain, Alain Paupe, Norbert Winer, and Yves Ville, "Endoscopic Laser Surgery versus Serial Amnioreduction for Severe Twin-to-Twin Transfusion Syndrome," *New England Journal of Medi-cine* 351, no. 2 (July 2004): 136–44, https://www.ncbi.nlm.nih.gov/pubmed /15238624.
8. See Rossi and D'Addario, "Survival Outcomes of Twin–Twin transfusion Syn-drome Stage I," Results section.

9. See Stephen P. Emery et al., "North American Fetal Therapy Network: Intervention vs. Expectant Management for Stage I Twin-Twin Transfusion Syndrome," *American Journal of Obstetrics and Gynecology* 215, no. 3 (September 2016): 346. e1–7, e1, https://pubmed.ncbi.nlm.nih.gov/27131587/.

10. See Khalil et al., "Evolution of Stage 1 Twin-to-Twin Transfusion Syndrome (TTTS)." The abstract for this article describes these findings without nuance, saying, "The optimal initial management of stage 1 TTTS remains in equipoise." The article describes its findings about Stage 1 TTTS as follows:

> The survival rates in the various subgroups, according to the management of stage 1 TTTS, do not show marked variation, but suggest that laser surgery as a first-line treatment might be associated with better survival. However, these results should be interpreted with caution as they are derived from observational data with their inherent risk of bias. The survival rates associated with amnioreduction or laser as the management of cases that had progressed, are likely to be worse than those which did not progress, so were managed expectantly, or in those pregnancies where laser surgery was performed, as a first-line treatment.

11. Ibid.

12. See Nassim Nicholas Taleb, *Black Swan: The Impact of the Highly Improbable* (New York: Random House, 2007).

13. See Khalil et al., "Evolution of Stage 1 Twin-to-Twin Transfusion Syndrome (TTTS)," Clinical and Research Implications of the Review Findings.

14. See U.S. National Library of Medicine, ClinicalTrials.gov, "Randomized Controlled Trial Comparing a Conservative Management and Laser Surgery (TTTS1)," NCT01220011 (July 20, 2020, update), http://clinicaltrials.gov/ct2/show/NCT01220011.

15. See Bamberg and Hecher, "Update on Twin-to-Twin Transfusion Syndrome," 58.

16. Simpson, "Twin-Twin Transfusion Syndrome," 7.

17. There were over 320,000 deaths from COVID-19 in the United States. See Johns Hopkins University, Coronavirus Resource Center, "COVID-19 United States Cases by County," https://coronavirus.jhu.edu/us-map.

18. See I. Couck, S. Ponnet, J. Deprest, R. Devlieger, L. De Catte, and L. Lewi, "Outcome of Selective Intrauterine Growth Restriction in Monochorionic Twin Pregnancies at 16, 20 or 30 Weeks according to the New Consensus Definition," *Ultrasound in Obstetrics and Gynecology* 56, no. 6 (December 2020): 821–30, https://doi.org/10.1002/uog.21975.

19. Ibid.

20. See F. G. Sileo, J. M. N. Duffy, R. Townsend, and A. Khalil, "Variation in Outcome Reporting across Studies Evaluating Interventions for Selective Fetal Growth Restriction," *Ultrasound in Obstetrics and Gynecology* 54 (2019): 101–5, 14, noting "sFGR in monochorionic diamniotic twin pregnancy is an uncommon condition with key differences from TTTS and other pathologies of monochorionic pregnancy that influence the outcomes investigated between these studies."

21. See Couck et al., "Outcome of Selective Intrauterine Growth Restriction," suppl. table S1: Details of Pregnancies with Selective Fetal Growth Restriction (sFGR) That Underwent Intervention, https://obgyn.onlinelibrary.wiley.com/action /downloadSupplement?doi=10.1002%2Fuog.21975&file=uog21975-sup-0001 -Supinfo.docx.

22. See Haruhiko Sago, Keisuke Ishii, Rika Sugibayashi, Katsusuke Ozawa, Masahiro Sumie, and Seiji Wada, "Fetoscopic Laser Photocoagulation for Twin–Twin Transfusion Syndrome," *Journal of Obstetrics and Gynaecology Research* 44, no. 5 (May 2018): 831–39, Amniotic Fluid Discordance and Selective Intrauterine Growth Restriction section, https://www.ncbi.nlm.nih.gov/pmc/articles /PMC5969296/.

23. See Ruben Quintero et al., "Neurodevelopmental Outcome of Monochorionic Twins with Selective Intrauterine Growth Restriction (SIUGR) Type II: Laser versus Expectant Management," *Journal of Maternal-Fetal and Neonatal Medicine* 34, no. 10 (2021): 1513–21, table 3, https://www.tandfonline.com/doi/full /10.1080/14767058.2019.1638902.

24. See Khalil et al., "Evolution of Stage 1 Twin-to-Twin Transfusion Syndrome (TTTS)," Clinical and Research Implications of the Review Findings.

25. Ibid.

26. See Spruijt et al., "Twin-Twin Transfusion Syndrome in the Era of Fetoscopic Laser Surgery," table 1.

27. See Fionnuala Mone, Barbara McConnell, Andrew Thompson, Ricardo Segurado, Peter Hepper, Moira C. Stewart, James C. Dornan, Stephen Ong, Fionnuala M. McAuliffe, and Michael D. Shields, "Fetal Umbilical Artery Doppler Pulsatility Index and Childhood Neurocognitive Outcome at 12 Years," *British Medical Journal Open* 6 (June 2016): e008916, https://www.ncbi.nlm.nih.gov /pmc/articles/PMC4916642/, describing "declarative memory" (the storage of facts and experiences that require conscious effort to recall).

28. Marojiln S. Spruijt, Enrico Lopriore, Ratna N. G. B. Tan, Femke Slaghekke, Frans J. C. M. Klumper, Johanna M. Middeldorp, Monique C. Haak, Dick

Oepkes, Monique Rijken, and Jeanine M. M. van Klink, "Long-Term Neuro-developmental Outcome in Twin-to-Twin Transfusion Syndrome: Is There Still Room for Improvement?," *Journal of Clinical Medicine* 8, no. 2 (2019): 1226, https://www.mdpi.com/2077-0383/8/8/1226.

29. See Bamberg and Hecher, "Update on Twin-to-Twin Transfusion Syndrome," 59–60.

30. Ibid.

31. See Suzanne L. Miller, Petra S. Huppi, and Carina Mallard, "The Consequences of Fetal Growth Restriction on Brain Structure and Neurodevelopmental Outcome," *Journal of Physiology* 594, no. 4 (January 2016): 807–23, https://pubmed.ncbi.nlm.nih.gov/26607046/.

32. See G. Favrais and E. Saliba, "Neurodevelopmental Outcome of Late-Preterm Infants: Literature Review," *Archives de Pédiatrie* 26 (November 2019): 492–96, 492, https://pubmed.ncbi.nlm.nih.gov/31704103/.

33. See Spruijt et al., "Twin-Twin Transfusion Syndrome in the Era of Fetoscopic Laser Surgery," Expert Opinion section.

34. See Vincenzo Berghella and Amanda Roman, "Cerclage in Twins: We Can Do Better!," *American Journal of Obstetrics and Gynecology* 211, no. 1 (July 2014): 5–6, https://www.ajog.org/article/S0002-9378(14)00247-6/fulltext.

35. See Amanda Roman, Noelia Zork, Sina Haeri, Corina N. Schoen, Gabriele Saccone, Sarah Colihan, Craig Zelig, Alexis C. Gimovsky, Neil S. Seligman, Fulvio Zullo, and Vincenzo Berghella, "Physical Examination-Indicated Cerclage in Twin Pregnancy: A Randomized Controlled Trial," *American Journal of Obstetrics and Gynecology* 223, no. 6 (December 2020): 902.e1–11, https://www.ajog.org/article/S0002-9378(20)30672-4/fulltext. But see an alternative conclusion that "twin pregnancies with a short cervix should not undergo cervical cerclage to reduce preterm delivery and adverse perinatal outcomes." Luis Sanchez-Ramos, "The Placement of a Cerclage in Patients with Twin Pregnancies and a Short Cervix Is Associated with Increased Risk of Preterm Birth and Adverse Perinatal Outcome," Letter to the Editor, *American Journal of Obstetric Gynecology* 222, no. 2 (February 2020): 194–96, https://doi.org/10.1016/j.ajog.2019.09.038.

36. See Spruijt et al., "Long-Term Neurodevelopmental Outcome in Twin-to-Twin Transfusion Syndrome," Discussion section.

37. Ibid.

38. See Sileo et al., "Variation in Outcome Reporting."

39. See C. Halling, F. D. Malone, F. M. Breathnach, M. C. Stewart, F. M. McAuliffe, J. J. Morrison, P. Dicker, F. Manning, J. D. Corcoran, and Perinatal Ireland Research Consortium, "Neuro-Developmental Outcome of a Large Cohort of

Growth Discordant Twins," *European Journal of Pediatrics* 175, no. 3 (October 2015): 381–89, https://europepmc.org/article/med/26490567.

40. See Maria Angela Rustico et al., "Selective Intrauterine Growth Restriction in Monochorionic Twins: Changing Patterns in Umbilical Artery Doppler Flow and Outcomes," *Ultrasound in Obstetrics and Gynecology* 49, no. 3 (2017): 387–93, https://pubmed.ncbi.nlm.nih.gov/27062653/.

41. See Sileo et al., "Variation in Outcome Reporting," 15. The same demonstration of the current lack of knowledge of the long-term outcomes of monochorionic twins with sIUGR was made by Sophie G. Groene, Lisanne S. A. Tollenaar, Dick Oepkes, Enrico Lopriore, and Jeanine M. M. van Klink, "The Impact of Selective Fetal Growth Restriction or Birth Weight Discordance on Long-Term Neurodevelopment in Monochorionic Twins: A Systematic Literature Review," *Journal of Clinical Medicine* 8, no. 7 (July 2019): 944, https://www.ncbi.nlm.nih.gov/pmc/articles/PMC6678939/.

42. See Ruben Quintero et al., "Neurodevelopmental Outcome of Monochorionic Twins with Selective Intrauterine Growth Restriction (SIUGR) Type II," Discussion section.

43. Ibid., table 1.

44. I did not encounter any study that indicated that the person pregnant with twins was other than a biological woman. Likewise, the studies did not note their subjects' gender presentation.

45. See Dongcai Wu, Linhuan Huang, Zhiming He, Xuan Huang, Qun Fan, and Yanmin Luo, "Preeclampsia in Twin Pregnancies: Association with Selective Intrauterine Growth Restriction," *Journal of Maternal Fetal Neonatal Medicine* 29, no. 12 (2016): 1967–71, doi:10.3109/14767058.2015.1070140.

46. See J. Duffy, M. Hirsch, L. Pealing, M. Showell, K. S. Khan, S. Ziebland, and R. J. McManus, "Inadequate Safety Reporting in Pre-Eclampsia Trials: A Systematic Evaluation," *British Journal of Obstetrics and Gynaecology* 125, no. 7 (June 2018): 795–803, 802, https://obgyn.onlinelibrary.wiley.com/doi/full/10.1111/1471-0528.14969.

47. See Sileo et al., "Variation in Outcome Reporting," 14.

48. Ibid.

49. See Adalina Sacco, Lennart Van der Veeken, Emma Bagshaw, Catherine Ferguson, Tim Van Mieghem, Anna L. David, and Jan Deprest, "Maternal Complications Following Open and Fetoscopic Fetal Surgery: A Systematic Review and Meta-Analysis," *Prenatal Diagnosis* 39, no. 4 (March 2019): 251–68, 251, https://obgyn.onlinelibrary.wiley.com/doi/full/10.1002/pd.5421.

50. Ibid.

51. Ibid., table 6: Long-Term Maternal Complications following Open and Feto-scopic Fetal Surgery.

52. Ibid., noting that the 95 percent confidence interval for psychological symptoms is 7.70–64.58.

53. See Simen Vergote, Liesbeth Lewi, Willem Gheysen, Luc De Catte, Roland Devlieger, and Jan Deprest, "Subsequent Fertility, Pregnancy, and Gynecologic Outcomes after Fetoscopic Laser Therapy for Twin-Twin Transfusion Syndrome Compared with Normal Monochorionic Twin Gestations," *American Journal of Obstetrics and Gynecology* 218, no. 4 (April 2018): 447.e1–7, Conclusion section, https://doi.org/10.1016/j.ajog.2018.01.013.

54. See Sacco et al., "Maternal Complications Following Open and Fetoscopic Fetal Surgery," 251.

55. See Ruth R. Faden and Tom L. Beauchamp, *A History and a Theory of Informed Consent* (New York: Oxford University Press, 1986).

56. Ibid., 304–5, describing the hypothetical cases of two pregnant women, Gretchen and Margaret, and the factors material to their choosing to have a C-section delivery.

57. Based on findings from the charmingly named TRUFFLE (Trial of Randomized Umbilical and Fetal Flow in Europe) study, the International Society of Ultra-sound in Obstetrics and Gynecology provided in August 2020 indicators for when a growth-restricted fetus should be delivered. See Christoph Lees, T. Stam-palija, A. A. Baschat, F. da Silva Costa, E. Ferrazzi, F. Figueras, K. Hecher, J. Kingdom, L. C. Poon, L. J. Salomon, and J. Unterscheider, "ISUOG Practice Guidelines: Diagnosis and Management of Small-for-Gestational-Age Fetus and Fetal Growth Restriction," *Ultrasound in Obstetrics and Gynecology* 56, no. 2 (August 2020): 298–312, https://obgyn.onlinelibrary.wiley.com/doi/full/10.1002/uog.22134.

58. See Christopher et al., "An Evidence-Based Approach to Determining Route of Delivery for Twin Gestations," 112.

59. See Daniel Grossman and Yanett Anaya, "The Myth of Ectopic Pregnancy Trans-plantation," BMJ Opinion (December 19, 2019), https://blogs.bmj.com/bmj/2019/12/17/the-myth-of-ectopic-pregnancy-transplantation/, describing two laws proposed in Ohio in 2019; neither piece of legislation was enacted.

60. See Elizabeth Chloe Romanis, "Is 'Viability' Viable? Abortion, Conceptual Confusion and the Law in England and Wales and the United States," *Journal of Law and Biosciences* 7, no. 1 (January–June 2020): 1–29, sec. vi, https://doi.org/10.1093/jlb/lsaa059, describing laws in Kansas, North Carolina, Texas, and

Wisconsin, which, absent contrary federal law, prohibit abortions after twenty weeks of gestation for any reason.

61. Medical providers are bound by medical ethics to provide information but may be required by law to provide falsehoods, such as stating, wrongly, that abortion increases breast cancer risk. See Callie Beusman, "A State-by-State List of the Lies Abortion Doctors Are Forced to Tell Women," Vice, August 18, 2016, https://www.vice.com/en/article/nz88gx/a-state-by-state-list-of-the-lies-abortion-doctors-are-forced-to-tell-women.

62. Crib bumpers have been tied to many infant fatalities. See Rachel Rabkin Peachman, "Proposed Ban on Padded Crib Bumpers by CPSC Will Save Lives," *Consumer Reports*, March 27, 2020, https://www.consumerreports.org/child-safety/ban-on-padded-crib-bumpers-cpsc/.

63. See Rachel Rabkin Peachman, "Guide to Recalled Infant Inclined Sleepers, Nappers, and Loungers," *Consumer Reports*, December 17, 2020, https://www.consumerreports.org/child-safety/recalled-infant-inclined-sleepers-nappers-loungers-guide/.

64. See Stephanie Zimmermann, "Despite Being Blamed in 50 Babies' Deaths, Inclined Infant Sleepers Available Online, Sun-Times Finds," *Chicago Sun-Times*, August 7, 2019, https://chicago.suntimes.com/2019/8/7/20757625/inclined-sleepers-infant-deaths-recalls-daycare-child-care-safety-consumer-kids-in-danger-us-pirg.

65. See Ashley Biviano, "Despite Fisher-Price Rock 'n Play Recall, Parents Say They'll Continue to Use the Sleeper," PressConnects.com, April 26, 2019, https://www.pressconnects.com/story/news/local/2019/04/26/fisher-price-rock-n-play-recall-refund-parents-continue-use-swing-babies/3574754002/.

66. See Rachel Rabkin Peachman, "While They Were Sleeping," *Consumer Reports*, December 30, 2019, https://www.consumerreports.org/child-safety/while-they-were-sleeping/.

67. See Peachman, "Guide to Recalled Infant Inclined Sleepers, Nappers, and Loungers."

68. See Ella Torres, "Parents Should Not Use Inclined Sleepers, Federal Agency Warns, Citing 73 Infant Deaths since 2005," ABC News, November 2, 2019, https://abcnews.go.com/US/parents-inclined-sleepers-federal-agency-warns-citing-73/story?id=66712626.

69. See Peachman, "Guide to Recalled Infant Inclined Sleepers, Nappers, and Loungers."

70. See Shankar Vedantam, "Facts Aren't Enough: The Psychology of False Beliefs," *Hidden Brain*, July 22, 2019, https://www.npr.org/transcripts/743195213,

interviewing Tali Sharot about the conclusions in her book, *The Influential Mind: What the Brain Reveals about Our Power to Change Others* (New York: Henry Holt, 2017).

71. Ibid.

72. See Clifford N. Lazarus, "Why Many People Stubbornly Refuse to Change Their Minds," *Psychology Today*, December 24, 2018, https://www.psychologytoday.com/us/blog/think-well/201812/why-many-people-stubbornly-refuse-change-their-minds.

73. See Jeremy Hobson, "How People Change Their Mind," *Here and Now*, WBUR-Boston, September 21, 2019, https://www.wbur.org/hereandnow/2018/09/21/how-people-change-their-mind, interviewing Hugo Mercier, cognitive scientist at the French National Center for Scientific Research and coauthor with Dan Sperber of *The Enigma of Reason*, about how people make up their minds—and how they change them.

74. See Elizabeth Kolbert, "Why Facts Don't Change Our Minds," Books, *New Yorker*, February 20, 2017, https://www.newyorker.com/magazine/2017/02/27/why-facts-dont-change-our-minds; also reviewing Hugo Mercier and Dan Sperber.

75. Ibid.

Epilogue

1. See CDC, "People with Certain Medical Conditions," COVID-19, December 28, 2020; updated May 13, 2021, https://www.cdc.gov/coronavirus/2019-ncov/need-extra-precautions/people-with-medical-conditions.html.

2. See CDC, "For Parents: Multisystem Inflammatory Syndrome in Children (MIS-C) Associated with COVID-19," May 20, 2020; updated February 24, 2021, https://www.cdc.gov/coronavirus/2019-ncov/daily-life-coping/children/mis-c.html.

3. See Ashley May, "Paid Family Leave Is an Elite Benefit in the U.S.," *USA Today*, May 17, 2017, https://www.usatoday.com/story/news/nation-now/2017/05/17/paid-maternity-leave-elite-benefit-u-s/325075001/.

4. See Catherine Pearson, "What the French Get So Right about Taking Care of New Moms," Huffington Post, January 17, 2017, https://www.huffpost.com/entry/what-the-french-get-so-right-about-taking-care-of-new-moms_n_587d27b4e4b086022ca939c4.

5. The Family Medical and Leave Act, which does not apply to my organization, requires that eligible employees receive twelve workweeks of unpaid leave in a

twelve-month period for the birth of a child and to care for the newborn child within one year of birth. See Wage and Hour Division, Department of Labor, "Family and Medical Leave Act," https://www.dol.gov/agencies/whd/fmla.

6. Although my employer was not bound by Obamacare's breastfeeding support provisions, as a health organization, it nevertheless provided generous and progressive support to nursing parents. Working a compressed schedule left me little time to take breast milk pumping breaks, however. I therefore expressed milk every three hours in my cubicle, hooking up my double pump under my shirt and continuing to peck away at my computer to the rhythmic sucking noise.

7. See Alan S. Brown, Catherine A. Schaefer, Richard J. Wyatt, Melissa D. Begg, Raymond Goetz, Michaeline A. Bresnahan, Jill Harkavy-Friedman, Jack M. Gorman, Dolores Malaspina, and Ezra S. Susser, "Paternal Age and Risk of Schizophrenia in Adult Offspring," *American Journal of Psychiatry* 159, no. 9 (September 2002): 1528–33, Discussion section, https://ajp.psychiatryonline.org/doi/full/10.1176/appi.ajp.159.9.1528.

8. See Connor Morrow Puleo, James Schmeidler, Abraham Reichenberg, Alexander Kolevzon, Latha V. Soorya, Joseph D. Buxbaum, and Jeremy M. Silverman, "Advancing Paternal Age and Simplex Autism," *Autism* 16, no. 4 (July 2012): 367–80, https://pubmed.ncbi.nlm.nih.gov/22180389/.

9. See Hanae Armitage, "Older Fathers Associated with Increased Birth Risks," Stanford Medicine News Center, October 31, 2018, https://med.stanford.edu/news/all-news/2018/10/older-fathers-associated-with-increased-birth-risks.html, describing the study by Yash S. Khandwala, Valerie L. Baker, Gary M. Shaw, David K Stevenson, Harold K. Faber, Ying Lu, and Michael L. Eisenberg, "Association of Paternal Age with Perinatal Outcomes between 2007 and 2016 in the United States: Population Based Cohort Study," *British Medical Journal* 363 (October 2018), Comparison with Other Studies section, https://www.bmj.com/content/363/bmj.k4372.

10. See Khandwala et al., "Association of Paternal Age with Perinatal Outcomes between 2007 and 2016 in the United States," Results section.

11. Ibid.

12. In fact, one Romanian study showed the opposite, that intrauterine grown restriction is more common for babies with younger fathers. See Monica G. Haşmaşanu, Sorana D. Bolboaca, Tudor C. Drugan, Melinda Matyas, and Gabriela C. Zaharie, "Parental Factors Associated with Intrauterine Growth Restriction," *Srpski Arhiv za Celokupno Lekarstvo* 143, no. 11–12 (November–December 2015): 701–6, https://pubmed.ncbi.nlm.nih.gov/26946765/.

13. "Arguably" because one study found older mothers are the more patient child caregivers, although no such finding was made for older fathers. I am unsurprised at these findings. See Tea Trillingsgaard and Dion Sommer, "Associations between Older Maternal Age, Use of Sanctions, and Children's Socio-Emotional Development through 7, 11, and 15 Years," *European Journal of Developmental Psychiatry* 15, no. 2 (December 2018): 141–55, https://www.tandfonline.com/doi/abs/10.1080/17405629.2016.1266248?journalCode=pedp20.

14. See K. Mac Dougall, Y. Beyene, and R. D. Nachtigall, "'Inconvenient Biology': Advantages and Disadvantages of First-Time Parenting after Age 40 Using *in vitro* Fertilization," *Human Reproduction* 27, no. 4 (April 2012): 1058–65, 1060, https://doi.org/10.1093/humrep/des007.

15. See M. Janecka, F. Rijsdijk, D. Rai, A. Modabbernia, and A. Reichenberg, "Advantageous Developmental Outcomes of Advancing Paternal Age," *Translational Psychiatry* 7 (June 2017): e1156, Discussion section, https://doi.org/10.1038/tp.2017.125, describing study of a large, nationally representative cohort of British twins and finding advantages of an older father for male children but little evidence of these advantages for female children.